Case Presentations for the MRCS and AFRCS

Titles in the series

Case Presentations in Accident and Emergency Medicine

Case Presentations in Anaesthesia and Intensive Care

Case Presentations in Arterial Disease

Case Presentations in Chemical Pathology

Case Presentations in Clinical Geriatric Medicine

Case Presentations in Clinical Infections

Case Presentations in Endocrinology and Diabetes

Case Presentations in Gastrointestinal Disease

Case Presentations in General Surgery

Case Presentations in Heart Disease (Second Edition)

Case Presentations in Medical Ophthalmology

Case Presentations for MRCS and AFRCS Volume 1

Case Presentations for MRCS and AFRCS Volume 2

Case Presentations for MRCS and AFRCS Volume 3

Case Presentations in Neurology

Case Presentations in Obstetrics and Gynaecology

Case Presentations in Otolaryngology

Case Presentations in Paediatrics

Case Presentations in Psychiatry

Case Presentations in Respiratory Medicine

Case Presentations in Urology

Case Presentations for the MRCS and AFRCS

Volume 3

Edited by

Philip Hornick BSc, MB BChir, FRCS
Lecturer, Department of Cardiothoracic Surgery,
Hammersmith Hospital, London

John Lumley MS, FRCS
Professor of Surgery, Professorial Surgical Unit,
St Bartholomew's Hospital, London

Pierce Grace MCh, FRCSI, FRCS
Professor of Surgical Science, University of Limerick,
Limerick

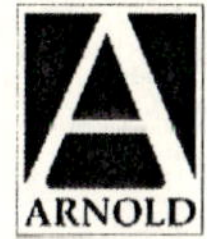

A member of the Hodder Headline Group
LONDON · NEW YORK · NEW DELHI

This edition first published in Great Britain in 1997 by Butterworth Heinemann.

This impression published by Arnold,
A member of the Hodder Headline Group,
338 Euston Road, London NW1 3BH

http://www.arnoldpublishers.com

Distributed in the USA by
Oxford University Press Inc.,
198 Madison Avenue, New York, NY10016
Oxford is a registered trademark of Oxford University Press

Whilst the advice and information in this book are believed to be true and accurate at the date of going to press, neither the authors nor the publisher can accept any legal responsibility or liability for any errors or omissions that may be made. In particular (but without limiting the generality of the preceding disclaimer) every effort has been made to check drug dosages; however, it is still possible that errors have been missed. Furthermore, dosage schedules are constantly being revised and new side-effects recognized. For these reasons the reader is strongly urged to consult the drug companies' printed instructions before administering any of the drugs recommended in this book.

British Library Cataloguing in Publication Data
A catalogue record for this book is available from the British Library

Library of Congress Cataloging-in-Publication Data
A catalog record for this book is available from the Library of Congress

ISBN 0 7506 3259 3

What do you think about this book? Or any other Arnold title?
Please send your comments to feedback.arnold@hodder.co.uk

Contents

Contributors

Terence J. Boyle BSc, FRCSI
Senior Registrar, Department of Surgery, University College Hospital, Galway, Ireland

Aubrey Bristow FRCA
Consultant Anaesthetist, St Bartholomew's Hospital, London

Paul Burke
Consultant Surgeon, Regional General Hospital, Limerick Ireland

L. Chadwick BA, BM, BCh, FRCS
Research Fellow and Honorary Registrar, Department of Neurosurgery, St Bartholomew's Hospital, London

Tom Creagh BSc, MCh, FRCSI
Consultant Urologist, Kingston Hospital, Kingston-upon-Thames

A.W. Darzi MD, FRCSI
Department of Surgery, Central Middlesex Hospital, London

David P. Drake MB BChir, FRCS, DCH
Consultant Surgeon, Department of Paediatric Surgery, Queen Elizabeth Hospital for Children, London

D.P. Dutka FRCP
Research Fellow and Honorary Senior Registrar, Department of Medicine (Clinical Cardiology), Royal Postgraduate Medical School, Hammersmith Hospital, London

John M. Fitzpatrick
Professor of Surgery, University College, Dublin; Consultant Urologist, Mater Misericordiae Hospital and University College Dublin, Ireland

George Geroulakos MD, FRCS, DIC, PhD
Lecturer in Surgery, Professorial Surgical Unit,
St Bartholomew's Hospital, London

Michael J. Gough MB, ChB, ChM, FRCS
Consultant Vascular Surgeon, The General Infirmary at Leeds, Leeds

Pierce Grace MCh, FRCSI, FRCS
Professor of Surgical Science, University of Limerick, Limerick, Ireland

P.J. Hamlyn BSc FRCS, MD
Consultant Neurosurgeon, St Bartholomew's Hospital, London

Charles Hinds FRCP, FRCA
Senior Lecturer and Consultant in Intensive Care, Intensive Care Unit, St Bartholomew's Hospital, London

Claire Hornick
Transplant Coordinator, North Thames East, Charterhouse Chambers, London

Pauline Jumaa MBBS, MSc, MRCPath
Senior Lecturer/Honorary Consultant, Department of Medical Microbiology, St Bartholomew's Hospital, London

M.J. Kelly MChir, FRCS, MRCP
Consultant Colorectal Surgeon, Leicester General Hospital, Leicester

K.P. Kumar MBBS, MS, FRCS
Vascular Surgical Unit, The General Infirmary at Leeds, Great George Street, Leeds

John Lumley MS, FRCS
Professor of Surgery, Professorial Surgical Unit,
St Bartholomew's Hospital, London

John A. Lynn MS, FRCS
Consultant Endocrine Surgeon, Hammersmith Hospital, London

Oliver J. McAnena MCh, FRCSI
Consultant Surgeon, Department of Surgery, University College Hospital, Galway, Ireland

Andrew McEvoy FRCS
Senior House Officer, Kingston Hospital, Kingston upon Thames

Averil O. Mansfield ChM, FRCS
Professor of Surgery, Academic Surgical Unit, St Mary's Hospital, London

Irwin Mohan FRCS
Senior House Officer in Surgery, St Mary's Hospital, London

Imran Mushtaq MB, ChB, FRCS
Registrar in Paediatric Surgery, Queen Elizabeth Hospital for Children, London

Charles C. Nduka BA, MB, BS(Hons)
Academical Surgical Unit, St Mary's Hospital, London

R. John Nicholls MChir, FRCS
St Mark's Hospital, Harrow, Middlesex

Michael O'Leary FRCA
Clinical Research Fellow in Intensive Care, St Bartholomew's Hospital, London

F.D. Opeyami Babatola MBBS, PhD, FRCA
Registrar, Department of Anaesthesia, Hammersmith Hospital, London

Geoffrey Raine FRCA, MB, ChB
Senior Registrar in Anaesthetics, Chelsea and Westminster Hospital, London

Lynn Riddell
Clinical Research Registrar, Department of Immunology, St Bartholomew's Hospital, London

Christopher John Rudge BSc, MBBS, FRCS
Consultant Transplant Surgeon, The Royal London Hospital, London

J.M. Ryan MCh, FRCS
The University College London Hospital, London

Charles Schamulian FRCA
Consultant Anaesthetist, Ealing Hospital, Middlesex

Humphrey Scott MS, FRCS
St Mark's Hospital, Harrow, Middlesex

David M. Scott-Coombes MS, FRCS
Senior Registrar in Surgery, Hammersmith Hospital, London

M. Sen FRCS(Eng)
Senior Registrar in Transplantation, St George's Hospital, London

Alastair Skelly BSc, MBBS, FRCA
Consultant and Honorary Senior Lecturer, Department of Anaestheisa, Hammersmith Hospital, London

Mark Smith BSc, MBBS, FRCA
Research Registrar, Department of Anaesthesia, Hammersmith Hospital, London

Martin Smith FRCA
Consultant Neuroanaesthetist, Tavistock Surgical Intensive Care Unit, The National Hospital for Neurology and Neurosurgery, London

Neil Soni MD, FANZCA
Director of Intensive Care, Chelsea and Westminster Hospital, London

Christopher T.M. Speakman MD, FRCS
St Mark's Hospital, Harrow, Middlesex

Gerard Stansby MChir, FRCS
Senior Lecturer/Honorary Consultant Surgeon, Academic Surgical Unit, St Mary's Hospital, London

Soad Tabaqchali FRCP, FRCPath
Professor, Clinical Director, Department of Medical Microbiology, St Bartholomew's Hospital, London

Jeremy N. Thompson, MChir, FRCS
Senior Lecturer/ Consultant Surgeon, Ealing and Hammersmith Hospitals, London

H.N. Whitfield MA, MCChir, FRCS
Department of Urology, Central Middlesex Hospital, London

D.A. Zideman QHP(C), BSc, MBBS, FRCA, Dip IMC
Consultant and Honorary Senior Lecturer, Department of Anaesthetics, Hammersmith Hospital, London

Preface

Postgraduate surgical training in the UK and Ireland has evolved to a new and more structured set point. The surgical colleges have introduced a number of new examinations – MRCS and AFRCS – to replace the old FRCS, which has become an intercollegiate exit examination. The new examinations specifically address surgical principles and practice and it is to the student approaching these written, oral and clinical assessments that this book is aimed. We chose the case history format as we consider it the most suitable and realistic medium for structured thought and clinically appropriate management.

When preparing for any examination, the candidate's continual wonder (and worry!) is 'what will they ask me?' and 'even if I know the answer, will it be enough?' To try and provide some insight into a prospective examiner's expectations we initially selected a broad range of topics from the syllabi of the new MRCS/AFRCS examinations. We then invited a large group of specialists, many of whom are examiners, to write case histories using a question-and-answer format at a level of knowledge that they would expect from a candidate for the MRCS/AFRCS exam. We asked that their histories be comprehensive, and to append a further reading list in order to provide the uninitiated reader with an overview, and an opportunity to read deeper into that particular condition. Their contributions, which emphasize basic surgical and scientific principles, form the basis of this book.

The mark of an expert is the ability to make one's own subject interesting and easily understood by everyone. This volume is a unique collection of surgical case histories written by experts for non-experts. The authors have done a magnificent job and we are delighted with the result. We hope that it will provide a flavour of the diversity of problems likely to be encountered during a lifetime in surgical practice, as well as indicating the 'height of the hurdles' which need to be jumped in order to pass the examinations. To the authors, on behalf of surgical examination candidates everywhere, we thank you.

P.H.
P.A.G.
J.S.P.L.

Acknowledgements

We would like to thank all the authors who have contributed so generously of their knowledge and time to this project. Without them this book would not exist.

We especially thank Mrs Vivienne Dignum, our literary co-ordinator, whose organization, enthusiasm and overall dedication made this book a reality.

Case 1 Thyroid nodule

One morning whilst shaving, a 24-year-old man noticed a lump in the lower part of his neck on the left side. He ignored it initially but after 2 weeks it had not disappeared and so he attended his general practitioner. She listened to him carefully and with the aid of a telephone call to the patient's mother elicited a history of radiotherapy to the neck in childhood for cervical lymphadenitis. On examination she found a hard painless solitary nodule in the thyroid gland and a serum thyroxine confirmed her clinical impression that he was euthyroid. She referred him urgently to a surgical outpatients.

Questions

1. What is the problem and what is the differential diagnosis?
2. How would you proceed to investigate this patient?
3. Classify the common neoplasms of the thyroid gland, describe the important features and discuss the treatment and prognosis.
4. What are the specific postoperative complications which may occur following thyroid surgery?

Answers

1. The problem is a solitary thyroid nodule and the differential diagnosis is given in Table 1.1.

Table 1.1 Differential diagnosis of a solitary thyroid nodule

Thyroid lesions	*Non-thyroid lesions*
Follicular adenoma*	Lymphadenopathy
Carcinoma*	Thyroglossal cyst
Colloid goitre*	Parathyroid adenoma
Cyst	Metastasis
Hashimoto thyroiditis	Carotid artery aneurysm
Lymphoma	

* The vast majority of thyroid nodules will be in these groups.

2

A solitary thyroid nodule can be felt in 4–7% of the population. The vast majority of such nodules are benign but about 5–10% of clinically significant thyroid nodules are malignant. In patients under 25 years of age, solitary nodules are neoplastic in about 50% of cases. A previous history of irradiation to the neck increases significantly the risk for later development of both malignant and benign lesions in the thyroid gland. Solitary nodules in men are more likely to be malignant than in women.

Non-thyroid lesions can usually be differentiated clinically from true thyroid lesions by the clinical observation that thyroid nodules move on swallowing. This occurs because the thyroid gland is invested by the pretracheal fascia and is attached firmly to the cricoid cartilage by the suspensory ligament of Berry. It is important to establish the thyroid status in a patient with a solitary nodule as nodules in a hyperactive thyroid are virtually never malignant.

2. Clinical assessment cannot differentiate between benign and malignant thyroid nodules. Scintiscanning (hypofunctioning nodules are more likely to be malignant) and ultrasonography (solid or mixed solid/cystic lesions are more likely to be neoplastic) have been used as the first line of investigation for many years but neither is very sensitive (i.e. detect all malignant lesions) or specific (i.e. all lesions detected are malignant). In recent years, fine-needle aspiration has become the investigation of choice for assessment of thyroid nodules and its use has reduced surgical exploration for thyroid nodules by 25%.

   The patient lies with a pillow supporting the shoulders to extend the neck. A 25-gauge needle is attached to a 10-ml syringe and under local anaesthetic the needle is introduced into the nodule. The plunger of the syringe is withdrawn to about the 8 ml mark and the needle is moved forwards and backwards for a distance of 1–2 mm within the nodule to disrupt the cells. As soon as liquid appears in the hub of the syringe, suction is released and the needle is withdrawn, and the contents of the needle are deposited on a slide that is immediately sprayed with alcohol for Papanicolaou staining. The procedure is repeated five times to sample different parts of the nodule.

3. Almost all neoplasms of the thyroid gland are epithelial in origin and are thus carcinomas. Most carcinomas arise from follicular epithelium and are classified histologically as

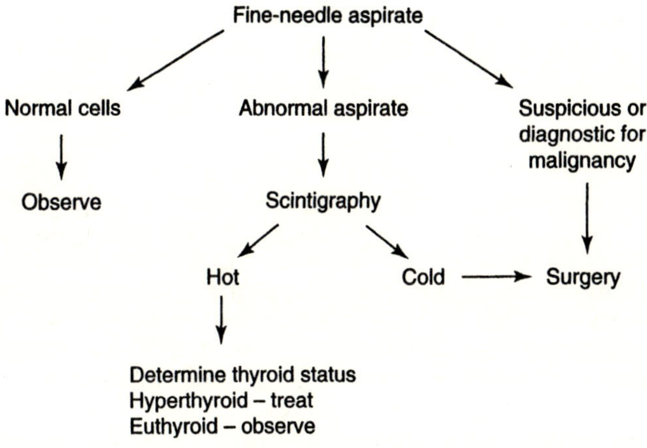

Figure 1.1 Algorithm for the management of a thyroid nodule.

papillary, follicular and anaplastic carcinomas. It is not unusual to have mixed papillary and follicular patterns. Medullary thyroid carcinoma arises from parafollicular (C-cell) elements and rarely is the thyroid the site of a metastasis or a fibro- or lymphosarcoma.

(a) *Papillary carcinoma* is the commonest type of thyroid cancer, accounting for 60% or more of cases. It occurs most often in young adults and in women more often than men. Most irradiation-induced thyroid cancers are papillary. They present as solitary nodules and most cases of occult thyroid cancer are papillary. They are slow-growing and metastasize via lymphatics to cervical nodes. Surgical treatment is controversial but lesions <2 cm in diameter should be treated by lobectomy. For larger lesions a total thyroidectomy on the affected side and a contralateral subtotal thyroidectomy should be performed. All patients should receive L-thyroxine to suppress thyroid stimulating hormone (TSH) post-operatively as TSH stimulates the growth of both papillary and follicular carcinoma. Patients with suspected secondaries should be evaluated for radioiodine therapy. The prognosis for patients with papillary thyroid cancer is excellent, even in the presence of lymph node metastases.

(b) *Follicular carcinoma* comprises about 20% of all malignant thyroid lesions. Its peak incidence is in the fourth decade and the sexes are equally affected. Follicular carcinoma may arise in a long-standing goitre or present as a solitary nodule. They are more malignant than papillary and metastases are usually haematogenous to bone, lung and liver. Surgery for follicular carcinoma consists of total lobectomy on the affected side and subtotal lobectomy on the contralateral side. As with papillary carcinoma, patients with follicular carcinoma should also be given L-thyroxine postoperatively to suppress TSH secretion. Systemic radioactive iodine (^{131}I) is used to destroy remaining thyroid tissue and metastases in patients with follicular carcinoma. To be effective, however, the patient has to be made hypothroid so that TSH levels will be high enough to promote ^{131}I concentration in the tissues.

Prognosis for patients with follicular carcinoma is worse than for papillary carcinoma and poor prognostic indicators include extrathyroid disease, distant metastases and older age.

(c) *Anaplastic carcinoma*, which accounts for 10% of thyroid cancers, occurs in older patients and slightly more often in women. They present as rapidly growing hard masses in the neck. They are very malignant with aggressive local invasion of skin, muscle, larynx, oesophagus and blood vessels. Usually no treatment is possible by the time the patient presents but surgery, radiotherapy and chemotherapy have all been tried with little success. Eighty per cent of patients are dead within a year of diagnosis.

(d) *Medullary thyroid carcinoma* comprises less than 5% of all thyroid cancers. It occurs after the age of 40 and is slightly more common in women. It metastazes to lymph nodes but also spreads haematogenously to lung, bone and liver. The important features of medullary thyroid carcinoma are:

(i) It arises from the parafollicular cells.
(ii) It secretes calcitonin, which can be used as a tumour marker.
(iii) It occurs in both sporadic and familial forms.
(iv) In the familial form it is associated with the multiple endocrine neoplasia (MEN) syndromes: MEN type

IIA (medullary thyroid carcinoma, phaeochromocytoma and hyperthyroidism) and MEN type IIB (medullary thyroid carcinoma, phaeochromocytoma, multiple mucosal neuromas, Marfanoid habitus and typical facies).

Treatment of medullary thyroid carcinoma should be undertaken only after a phaeochromocytoma has been sought (24-h urinary vanillylmandelic acid and computed tomographic scan) and treated or excluded. Treatment is by surgery alone, which consists of a total thyroidectomy because of the high incidence of multicentric lesions with removal of surrounding soft tissues and nodes, particularly in the central part of the neck. Neither hormone nor radioiodine therapy is indicated in the management of medullary carcinoma.

Prognosis is slightly worse than follicular carcinoma, with an overall 5-year survival of about 50%. However, operative treatment in the absence of metastases is usually curative. Other family members should be screened for phaeochromocytoma.

4. (a) *Haemorrhage* is usually reactionary and occurs in the first 24 h after surgery. Major bleeding may arise from failure to secure the superior thyroid vessels, the inferior thyroid artery or the thyroid veins. An accumulating haematoma will cause respiratory obstruction and a patient who has stridor postoperatively requires immediate evacuation of the wound, and this may need to be performed at the bedside. The wound should then be re-explored and the bleeding site secured. Suture ligatures are less likely to become dislodged than simple ligatures and this technique should be employed for all vessels in the neck.

(b) *Recurrent laryngeal nerve damage* occurs in about 0.2% of thyroidectomies. Prior to surgery, indirect laryngoscopy should be performed to ensure that both vocal cords are moving normally. Patients with neoplasms may have recurrent laryngeal involvement although usually these patients will be hoarse. During surgery the recurrent laryngeal nerves should be identified and preserved. Bilateral recurrent laryngeal nerve injury is a devastating complication. The patient is unable to speak and the least exertion causes airway obstruction.

Immediate treatment is by tracheostomy and subsequently arytenoidectomy may be performed to hold the airway open.

(c) *Superior laryngeal nerve (external branch) damage* is characterized by a loss of pitch and inability to make explosive sounds. The true incidence of this complication is unknown but it may occur in up to 25% of patients. However, it is usually transient.

(d) *Hypoparathyroidism* occurs in about 8% of patients following thyroidectomy. The serum calcium should be checked routinely postoperatively. Hypoparathyroidism usually presents within a week of surgery and should be treated initially with oral calcium 2–3 g/day and vitamin D (calciferol 25 000–100 000 units/day) if hypocalcaemia persists in spite of calcium supplementation.

(e) *Hypothyroidism* always occurs after total thyroidectomy and in about 15% of patients following subtotal thyroidectomy for Graves disease.

(f) *Thyroid storm or crisis* is now a very rare complication of thyroidectomy. It occurs following surgery on thyrotoxic patients but other events, e.g. pneumonia, can precipitate a crisis in hyperthyroid patients. Clinically a thyroid crisis presents with confusion, delirium leading to coma, high fever and severe tachycardia (130–200 beats/min). Treatment is aimed at rapid control of thyrotoxicosis by administration of antithyroid drugs (propylthiouracil or methimazole and iodine) and blocking the peripheral actions of the hormone by administering beta blockers. Supportive therapy, including intravenous fluids, cooling for hyperthermia (aspirin should not be used) and diuretics and digoxin for heart failure should also be instituted.

Further reading

Lynn J and Bloom SR. (1993) *Surgical Endocrinology*, Butterworth-Heinemann, Oxford

Pierce Grace

Case 2 Fat embolism

Male 27 years	Weight 74 kg
Reason for admission:	Fractured femur following a motor cycle accident Was unconscious for approximately 5 min but on admission to hospital was fully lucid with a Glasgow Coma Scale of 15
Medical history:	Smokes 30 cigarettes/day Alcohol – 20 beers/week Amateur body builder
Progress:	Was taken to theatre for a pinning of a femur. During the operation was given 2 units of blood. Recovery was uneventful. Three days later suddenly developed chest pain and collapsed. He was rapidly and easily resuscitated. Transferred to intensive therapy unit (ITU)
On admission to ITU:	Blood pressure 110/70 mmHg Pulse rate 100 beats/min Temperature 38°C Retinal petechiae Chest X-ray normal Blood gases: pH 7.14 P_{CO_2} 8.4 kPa P_{O_2} 9.0 kPa oxygen saturation 99% Base excess −8.4 mmol/l on 60% oxygen
After 24 hours:	Blood pressure 78/44 mmHg Pulse rate 120 beats/min regular Temperature 39.4°C Chest X-ray showed bilateral fluffy shadows Blood cultures: *Staphyococcus aureus*

Questions

1. What was the likely cause of his initial collapse?
2. What is the pathophysiology of this condition?
3. What must you exclude from the diagnosis?
4. What are the signs and symptoms and how would you attempt to confirm the diagnosis?
5. What happened after 24 h and what is the most likely cause?
6. What are the routes leading to nosocomial infections?
7. What are the predisposing factors?
8. What are the principles of management of:
   (a) Fat embolus?
   (b) Noscomial infections?

Answers

1. Fat embolus.
2. Fat emboli originate from exposed marrow at the site of the fracture. Large fat cells are injured, releasing smaller fat globules. These then gain access to the circulation via torn venules within the marrow substances (Fig. 2.1).

   The fat emboli become coated with platelets which will then release a number of mediators. These will result in bronchospasm, ventilation–perfusion mismatch, leading to capillary congestion, oedema, hypoxemia, hypoperfusion and ultimately cellular damage with the release of tissue lipases. The lipases will then act on the fat emboli, releasing free fatty acids (FFAs) and glycerol. These FFAs, together with the increase in circulating FFAs which result from the stress of the trauma (due to the effect of catecholamines on fat), will result in lung damage McNamara *et al.* (1972).

   The presence of a petechial rash implies that fat emboli have gained access to the arterial circulation. This is probably via alveolar capillaries or precapillary shunts which have opened due to the increased arterial pressure.

   The cerebral histological features consist of widespread petechial haemorrhages throughout the white matter of the cortex and, to a lesser extent, the brainstem and spinal cord. Lipases will then act on the FFAs in the brain, with resultant encephalopathy and neurological deficits.

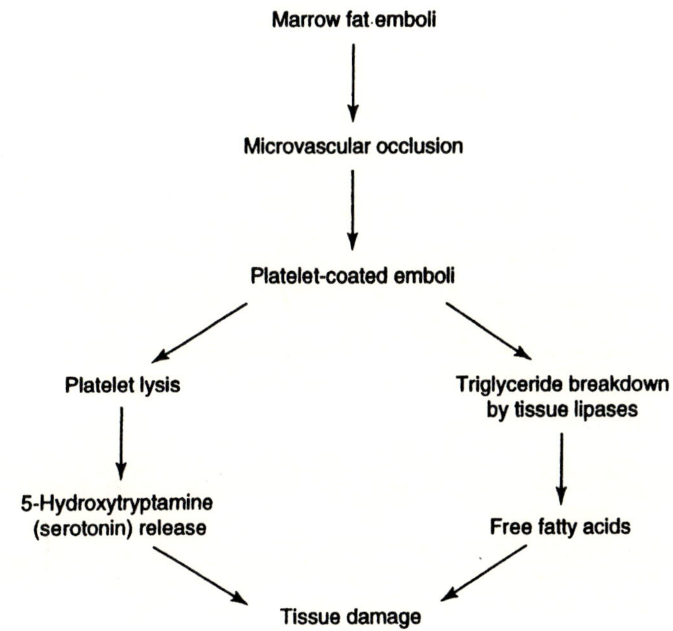

Fig. 2.1 Pathophysiology of the fat embolism syndrome. From van Besouw and Hinds (1989), with permission.

3. (a) Subdural haematoma.
   (b) Damage to the aorta, especially at the origin of the left subclavian artery.
   (c) Tear of the oesophagus.
4. The diagnosis is based on both biochemical and clinical features (Table 2.1; Gurd and Wilson, 1974).

   However, it has been found that tachycardia, tachypnoea, pyrexia and central nervous system involvement in the presence of arterial hypoxia are better indicators (Murray and Racz, 1974).

   A fat embolus index has been suggested by Schonfeld *et al.* (1983). A positive diagnosis can be made if there is a cumulative score of over 5 (Table 2.2).

   A diagnosis based solely on respiratory parameters has been advocated (Lindeque *et al.*, 1987). Only one single criterion together with a long bone fracture is considered

Table 2.1 Criteria for diagnosis of fat embolism

Major features
Respiratory insufficiency
Cerebral signs
Petechial rash
Minor features
Pyrexia
Tachycardia
Retinal involvement
Jaundic
Renal involvement
Fat macroglobulinaemia

The presence of one major and four minor features and fat macroglobulinaemia is diagnostic.
From Gurd and Wilson (1974), with permission.

diagnostic, however, this probably leads to over-diagnosis of fat embolus:

(a) Sustained $Pa\text{O}_2$ <8.0 kPa.
(b) Sustained $Pa\text{CO}_2$ <7.5 kPa or pH <7.3.
(c) Respiratory rate >35 breaths/min.

(a) *Respiratory insufficiency.* This occurs in 75% of patients, commonly 2–3 days after injury.
 The effects on the lung occur in two phases:
 (i) The first is immediate, due to mechanical obstruction of the pulmonary vessels.
 (ii) The second phase occurs when chemical pneumonitis develops. The capillary endothelium becomes

Table 2.2 Diagnosis of fat embolism syndrome using a fat embolism index

Symptom	*Score*
Petechiae	5
Diffuse alveolar infiltrates	4
Hypoxaemia ($Pa\text{O}_2$ <9.3 kPa)	3
Confusion	1
Fever >38°C	1
Heart rate >120 beats/min	1
Respiratory rate >30 breaths/min	1

From Lindeque *et al.* (1987), with permission.

inflamed as the result of breakdown of fat globules into toxic FFAs and from the release of serotonin and histamine from platelets and mast cells. Exudation across the pulmonary capillary endothelium occurs, with intra-alveolar haemorrhage (Oh, 1985).

The clinical signs are of dyspnoea, tachypnoea, chest pains and fine inspiratory crackles. The chest X-ray may at first be normal but, as the condition worsens, bilateral fluffy shadows develop – the classical snow storm appearance (Arthurs *et al.*, 1993).

Hypoxaemia is one of the earliest signs and usually precedes respiratory distress by a number of hours (Schlag *et al.*, 1993).

In all, 10% of patients will develop acute respiratory distress syndrome.

(b) *Cerebral features.* These are due to systemic emboli and occur in 86% of patients (Van Besouw and Hinds, 1989) and can precede the respiratory symptoms by 6–12 h. It is postulated that fat globules enter the systemic circulation through the pulmonary capillaries, arteriovenous shunts or a patent foramen ovale (Oh, 1985). Released thromboplastin induces platelet aggregation on to fat globules. Central nervous system microvascular thrombosis ensues. Patients thus develop an encephopathy which is aggravated by hypoxaemia but which is not alleviated by oxygen therapy.

In some patients, diverse focal neurological symptoms can occur, e.g. hemiplegia, apraxia, aphasia, scotomata and conjugate deviation of the eyes.

Computed tomography is of little help in diagnosing the FES but does help to exclude other possible causes of focal lesions, such as subdural haematoma.

(c) *Dermatological features.* These occur in 60% of patients and are due to fat emboli within the dermal capillaries. This produces a petechial rash within 36 h (Haplan *et al.*, 1986), which is most marked over the conjunctivae, oral mucous membrane and skin folds of the upper half of the body, particularly the neck and axillae. The rash usually resolves within 7 days.

(d) *Other features*

(i) Non-specific pyrexia and tachycardia, which may be associated with a superimposed infection.

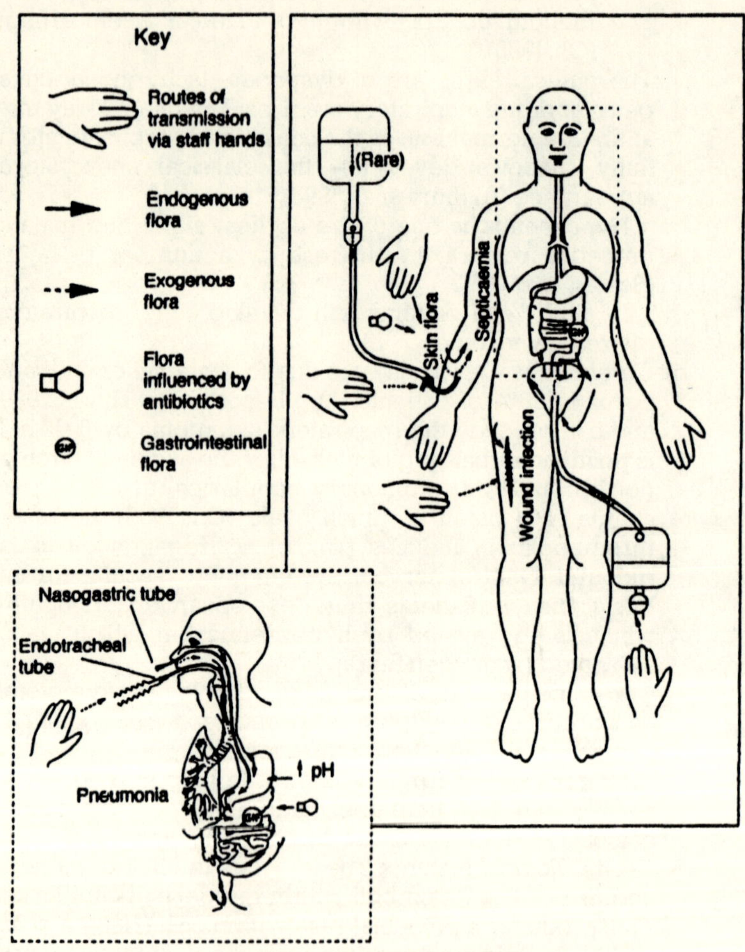

Fig. 2.2 The common pathways by which the nosocomial bacteria that cause sepsis in the intensive therapy unit may enter the patient.

  - (ii) Electrocardiogram changes may show signs of right ventricular strain.
  - (iii) Retinal changes include soft fluffy exudates, macular oedema and retinal haemorrhage.
  - (iv) Renal changes may present with oliguria, lipuria, proteinuria or haematuria, which is usually short-lived.
  - (v) Jaundice is rare and generally self-limiting.
- (e) *Laboratory investigations*
  - (i) Decrease in haemoglobin.
  - (ii) Decrease in platelets.
  - (iii) Increase in fibrinogen degradation products.
  - (iv) Increase in the prothrombin time.
  - (v) Increase in the thrombin time.
  - (vi) Increase in the erythrocyte sedimentation rate.
  - (vii) Fat macroglobulinaemia.
  - (viii) Decrease in serum calcium because of an affinity of calcium ions for FFAs.
  - (ix) Increase in FFAs.
  - (x) Sputum, urine and cerebrospinal fluid may stain positive for fat.
  - (xi) Increase in cortisol.
  - (xii) Increase in glucagon.
  - (xiii) Increase in cathecholamines.
  - (xiv) Decrease in serum albumin, probably due to an increase in capillary permeability.

  The last four are directly related to the stress response.

5. The patient became septic, probably as a result of acquiring a nosocomial infection.
6. Nosocomial infections are infections acquired in hospital. The sources of nosocomial infections are illustrated in Figure 2.2 (Baxter, 1994).
   - (a) *Source*
     - (i) Environmental: from ward dust, e.g. *Staphylococcus aureus*, and from humidified water, e.g. *Pseudomonas aeruginosa*.
     - (ii) Patients and staff: endogenous flora, e.g. *P. aeruginosa* from gut flora, and exogenous flora, e.g. *Klebsiella aerogenes* colonizing the patient's skin.

(b) *Routes of transmission*

(i) Hands: indirectly via infected gloves (by the environment) and directly via the nose and skin of staff, e.g. *S. aureus.*

(ii) Air: from patients and staff, e.g. *Streptococcus pneumoniae*; from ventilator tubing, i.e. Enterobacteriaceae; from dust in surgical wounds; from air-conditioning equipment, e.g. *Legionella.*

(iii) Common vehicle: episodic, e.g. due to inadequate sterilization of reusable instruments, and epidemic, e.g. contamination of intravenous fluids and drugs.

(iv) Portal of entry: skin, via intravenous cannulae and surgical wounds; inhalational via contaminated water from humidifiers; ingestion via contamination of enteral feeds; urinary tract via urinary catheter.

7. (a) *In nosocomial pneumonia*

(i) Endotracheal intubation is the single most important risk factor.

(ii) Elderly patients are especially at risk.

(iii) It is encouraged by the administration of broad-spectrum antibiotics.

(iv) Administration of H_2-blockers leads to alkalization and bacterial colonization of the stomach and microaspiration.

(b) *In nosocomial septicaemia*

(i) Urinary tract infection rarely leads to septicaemia.

(ii) Septicaemia is usually associated with intravenous devices (puncture site, taps and parenteral fluid).

(iii) Septicaemia may also arise from skin flora, infusion equipment and flora from the hands of staff.

8. (a) *Fat embolus.* The first aim is to attempt specifically to treat the consequences of the fat itself:

(i) Alcohol – this will inhibit lipase activity and thus decrease FFA production. However, its efficacy is not proven.

(ii) Heparin (2500 units 6-hourly) will increase lipase activity and thus will reduce the amount of circulating fat globules. However, it has the potential of increasing FFAs and its efficacy is also not proven.

(iii) Low-molecular-weight dextran (dextran 40) will reduce red cell aggregation, expand plasma volume, decrease blood viscosity and reduce platelet stickiness. There is little convincing practical evidence that it works, and it does have the potential to effect coagulation and can produce renal failure, especially in hypovolaemic patients.

All the above therefore show little convincing proof of producing any benefit and are not recommended.

(iv) *Aprotinin.* This is a protease inhibitor. It has been shown to decrease the mortality rate from 15% to 5%. However, no well-designed trials have confirmed these results. The results of trials in progress are eagerly awaited as it appears that aprotinin may be of benefit.

(v) *Steroids.* Mainly methylprednisilone (7.5 mg/kg 6-hourly for 12 doses) is postulated to stabilize membranes, limit the amount of FFAs produced and inhibit complement-mediated leukocyte aggregation (Schonfeld *et al.*, 1983). However, for steroids to be effective they probably need to be given early and as a prophylactic measure.

(vi) *Albumin.* Experimentally it has been shown that albumin binds FFAs, thus making them non-toxic. Large amounts of albumin are required as their binding sites are rapidly saturated with the large numbers of FFAs produced in the acute phase.

Supportive measures

(i) Aggressive correction of the hypoxaemia using continuous positive airway pressure or intermittent mandatory ventilation if necessary.

(ii) Conscientious attention to fluid and electrolyte balance.

(iii) Correction of anaemia.

(iv) Early mobilization appears to decrease the amount of fat released into the circulation.

(b) *Nosocomial infections*

(i) Treating patients with antibiotic or antifungal agents. As a basic principle, one should try and identify the organism, ascertain its susceptibility and treat it with an antimicrobial agent which has the narrowest spectrum of activity. This is to try and prevent superinfection and resistance developing.

If an organism cannot be identified and if the sepsis syndrome ensues, it is then justified to use an agent with activity against Gram-negative, Gram-positive and anaerobic bacteria. In this regard Tazocin and imipenem are of value.

It has been suggested that local antibiotic strategies applied to the nose and oropharynx may help decrease the incidence of nosocomial pneumonia. This is very time-consuming and expensive and it is questionable whether the ends justify the means (van Uffelen *et al.*, 1987).

Removing humidifiers from ventilator circuits and replacing them with thin pleated membrane filters should be seriously considered. These filters have been shown to humidify the air by up to 28–32 mg H_2O/l (Chalon *et al.*, 1984). More importantly, they will filter up to 99.999% of air-borne bacteria and 100% of liquid-borne bacteria (Hedley and Allt-Graham, 1992).

(ii) Removing the infected material. Any obvious sites of infection should either be excised or drained. Lines should be changed every 4–5 days. Scrupulous hygiene should be maintained during endotracheal suction. Staff should ensure that gloves are changed regularly.

(iii) Support failing organ systems: use ventilation, fluid therapy, vasodilators, inotropes and parenteral nutrition.

More recent therapies are being directed towards the inflammatory protein mediators (Cohen, 1994):

Monoclonal antibodies against endotoxin.

Cloned fragments from bactericidal/permeability factor.

Soluble CD14 as an endotoxin-neutralizing agent.

sTNFR-IgG binds avidly to tumour necrosis factor.

Interleukin-1 receptor antagonist against interleukin-1.

Regulatory cytokines that down-regulate the immune system, i.e. interleukin-10 (Gerard *et al.*, 1993).

Attempts have been made to inhibit the production and also the effects of induced nitric oxide (Cobb *et al.*, 1993).

To date these newer therapies have met with rather limited success and at present they remain research tools. There can be no doubt that as our knowledge of inflammatory proteins improves and as nitric oxide research expands, newer and more useful therapies will become available in our fight against these major causes of death in intensive care.

References and further reading

Arthurs MH, Morgan C and Sivapragasam S. (1993) Fat embolism syndrome following long bone fractures. *W.I. Medical Journal* **42:** 115–117

Balk RA and Bone RC. (1989) The septic syndrome: definition and clinical implications. *Critical Care Clinics* **5:** 1–8

Baxter C. (1994) *American Journal of Surgery* **167** (suppl. 1A): 12–14

Chalon J. Markham J, Ali MA and Ramanathan S. (1984) The pall Ultipor breathing circuit filter- and efficient heat and moisture exchanger. *Anesthesia and Analgesia* **63:** 566–570

Cobb JP, Cunnion RE and Danner RL. (1993) Nitric oxide as a target for therapy in septic shock. *Critical Care Medicine* **21:** 1261–1263

Cohen J (1994) Novel pharmacological approaches to sepsis. *Current Opinions in Anaesthesia* **7:** 141–145

Drugs and Therapeutics Bulletin (1994) **32:** 91–96

Gerard C, Bruyns C, Marchant A *et al.* (1993) Interleukin 10 reduces the lethality of tumour necrosis factor and prevents lethality. *Journal of Experimental Endoxtoxemia* **177:** 547–550

Gurd AR and Wilson RI (1974) The fat embolism syndrome. *Journal of Bone and Joint Surgery* **56B:** 408–416

Haplan RP, Grant JM and Kaufman AJ. (1986) Dermatologic features of fat embolism syndrome. *Cutis* **38:** 52–55

Hawkey P and Bodenham A. (1900) *Sepsis in the Intensive Therapy Unit. The Bayer Anti-infective Lecture Notes Series.* Franklin Scientific Projects

Hedley RM and Allt-Graham J. (1992) A comparison of the filtration properties of heat and moisture exchangers. *Anaesthesia* **47:** 414–420

Hillhouse E. (1994) Cell signaling: key roles of nitric oxide and neuropeptides. *Hospital Update* 462

Hoeft A and Mann D. (1994) Myocardial dysfunction in septic shock. *COIA* **7:** 26–32

Landlow L and Anderson W. (1994) Splanchnic ischaemia and its role in multi organ failure. *Acta Anaesthesiologica Scandinavica* **38:** 626–639

Lindeque BG, Schoeman HS, Domisse GF, Boeyens MC and Vlok AL. (1987) Fat embolism and the fat embolism syndrome: a double blind therapeutic study. *Journal of Bone Joint Surgery* **69:** 128–131

McNamara JD, Molat M, Dunn R, Burran EL and Stremple JF. (1972) Lipid metabolism after trauma. *Journal of Thoracic Cardiovascular Surgery* **60:** 968–972

Marino PL. (1991) *The ICU Book.* Lea & Febiger, Philadelphia

Murray DG and Racz GB. (1974) Fat embolism syndrome (respiratory insufficiency syndrome). A rationale for treatment. *Journal of Bone and Joint Surgery* **56A:** 1338–1349

Oh TE. (1985) Fat embolism. In: *Intensive Care Manual,* 2nd edn, Oh TE (ed.) Butterworth-Heinemann, Oxford, pp. 110 122

Redl H and Schlag G. (1994) ARDS – mediators of inflammation. *Current Opinions in Anaesthesiology* **7:** 146–152

Schlag G, Redl H, Baharami S, Davies J, Smuts P and Marzi I. (1993) Trauma and cytokines. In: *Shock, Sepsis and Organ failure. Cytokine Network*, 1st edn, Schlag G, Redl H and Taber DL (eds). Springer-Verlag, Berlin, pp. 128–162

Schonfeld SA, Ploysongsang Y, DiLisio R *et al.* (1983) Fat embolism prophylaxis with corticosteroids. *Annals of Internal Medicine* **99:** 438–443

Vallance P and Collier J (1994) Biology and clinical relevance of nitric oxide. *British Medical Journal* **309:** 453–457

Van Besouw JP and Hinds CJ (1989) Fat embolism syndrome. *British Journal of Hospital Medicine* **42:** 304–311

van Uffelen R, Rommes JH and van Saene HKF. (1987) Preventing lower airway colonisation and infection in mechanically ventilated patients. *Critical Care Medicine* **15:** 99–102

Charles Schamulian

Case 3 Head injury

A 44-year-old man attends the accident and emergency department of his local hospital, having been hit over the head accidentally with a golf club whilst playing a round. He did not lose consciousness and is oriented with no neurological signs. He does, however, have a 3-cm laceration on his forehead just in front of the hairline and on palpation a dent is thought to be felt in the underlying bone.

Questions

1. What investigations are necessary to confirm the diagnosis and aid in its management?
2. How should this condition be managed?
3. Describe the indications for surgery for closed depressed skull fractures.
4. What is a growing skull fracture and how is it managed?
5. What are the important complications of a compound depressed skull fracture?
6. What is the management of cerebrospinal fluid (CSF) rhinorrhoea and what are the indications for antibiotic prophylaxis in head injuries?

Answers

1. Plain skull X-rays, anteroposterior and lateral views, are necessary. Depressed fractures viewed *en face* cause a double density as a result of the overlap of bone. Tangential views may be required to delineate the depressed fracture completely. A skull fracture is defined as depressed if the outer table of one or more of the fractured segments lies below the level of the inner table of the surrounding intact skull.

   If a depressed fracture is confirmed, a computed tomographic (CT) scan should be performed (both on brain and bony windows) to determine the extent of the depression, whether the dura is torn (sometimes air can be seen within the cranial vault), whether there is any underlying brain injury and associated pathology, such as a haematoma, and whether there is involvement of the air sinuses.

2. Surgery should proceed as early as possible and within 24 h. The wound should be debrided and the bone fragments elevated, cleaned and replaced as much as possible. A tear in the dura should be sutured and any underlying necrotic brain should be removed. Antibiotic prophylaxis should be given to prevent abscess formation. If one of the air sinuses is extensively involved in the fracture, it may need to be formally obliterated and a craniofacial repair performed. The exception to this surgical management is if the fracture is over one of the major venous sinuses, when attempts at elevation can lead to catastrophic bleeding. In these cases the patient should just be treated with antibiotics.
3. In adults, simple depressed skull fractures may often be left alone, with one of the main indications for surgery being cosmesis. In very young children even large depressions can be left alone, as when the skull grows it remoulds itself to reduce the size of the defect. However, if there is a dural tear in young children some surgeons advocate operating prophylactically to prevent a growing skull fracture. Other indications for surgery in adults are if the radiological appearances suggest a dural tear, and if there is any underlying brain pathology or haematoma formation. Also, if the fracture involves the air sinuses it should be treated as a compound fracture.
4. A growing skull fracture occurs in infants and very young children who have previously suffered a traumatic skull fracture associated with a dural tear. Rarely, it may occur in adults. The patient presents months or years afterwards, with a cranial mass at the site of the fracture which is soft, pulsatile and may transilluminate. Plain skull X-rays show a bony defect in the course of a skull fracture, whose margins are irregular with a wavy, scalloped contour. The majority of growing fractures occur in the parietal region. The mass is the arachnoid membrane projecting through the dural tear containing CSF, and occasionally brain. There must be some form of valve mechanism present allowing free entry of CSF into the arachnoid sac but inhibiting its return. Without treatment the mass may continue to enlarge in size, further eroding the bone and occasionally causing a neurological deficit. The basis of treatment is surgery with the aim of repairing the dural and bony defects.

5. If there is a compound fracture tearing the dura there is a risk of the patient developing meningitis or a cerebral abscess, particularly if surgery has been delayed for any reason or is inadequate. Even with prompt and adequate surgery, wound infections will occur in 5–10% of cases.

   The incidence of seizures depends on the presence or absence of a dural tear. Whilst early epilepsy after a depressed fracture occurs in 8% with the dura intact and 11% if the dura is torn, late epilepsy occurs in 24% if the dura is torn, but only 7% if the dura is intact. Many surgeons prescribe anticonvulsants prophylactically if there is a dural tear, and others to all cases of depressed skull fracture. Most patients however, have their anticonvulsants stopped in the postoperative period, and are only given them long-term if they actually fit. Surgery does not alter the incidence of epilepsy.

   If bone replacement has been inadequate due to a loss of bone during the injury or all of the bone is too contaminated to replace, there may still be a cosmetic defect when all the swelling has disappeared. In this case the patient will need a cranioplasty using his or her own ribs, acrylic resin or a titanium plate. The cranioplasty should be delayed for 6–12 months after the initial surgery to minimize the risk of infection.
6. The management of CSF rhinorrhoea is controversial. The conservative view is that most leaks will stop in 7–10 days, and the patient should be observed during this time. Traditionally antibiotic prophylaxis is given during the period of the leak; however, recently some surgeons feel that the use of antibiotics just encourages the occurrence of antibiotic-resistant meningitis. Often surgery is only contemplated if the CSF leak continues for more than 14 days. However, the alternative view is that, even if the leak stops, the patient is at risk of developing meningitis at any time in the future because the dural defect may have been plugged by herniated brain. Thus surgery is advocated in all cases.

   In general, antibiotics should only be used if there is a communication between the intradural structures and the external environment. These cases for antibiotics in a compound fracture and rhinorrhoea have been dealt with above. If an intracranial pressure monitor is being used, antibiotics are given for the duration of time the monitor is in place.

Further reading

Becker DP, Gade GF, Young HF and Feurman TF. (1990) Diagnosis and treatment of head injury in adults. In: *Neurological Surgery*, 3rd edn, vol 3, Youmans JR (ed.). WB Saunders, Philadelphia, pp. 2017–2148

Eljamel MSM and Foy PM. (1990) Post-traumatic CSF fistulae, the case for surgical repair. *British Journal of Neurosurgery* **4:** 479–483

Jennett B, Miller JD and Braakman R. (1974) Epilepsy after nonmissile depressed skull fracture. *Journal of Neurosurgery* 41: 208–216

L. Chadwick
P.J. Hamlyn

Case 4 Splenic trauma

A 17-year-old male was kicked in the lower left chest by a horse. On arrival in the accident and emergency department 1 h after the injury, the patient was haemodynamically stable (blood pressure 130/60 mmHg; pulse 75 beats/min). He complained of pain at the site of injury to his ribcage, and also of left shoulder pain, particularly on inspiration. Chest X-ray was normal; specifically there were no rib fractures. A full blood count revealed a haemoglobin of 11 g/dl. Diagnostic peritoneal lavage was positive for blood. The extent of splenic injury was assessed using computed tomography (CT; Fig. 4.1). Two hours following his arrival the patient developed a persistent tachycardia with hypotension. Attempted conservative management with intravenous fluid resuscitation failed and he underwent a laparotomy and splenectomy.

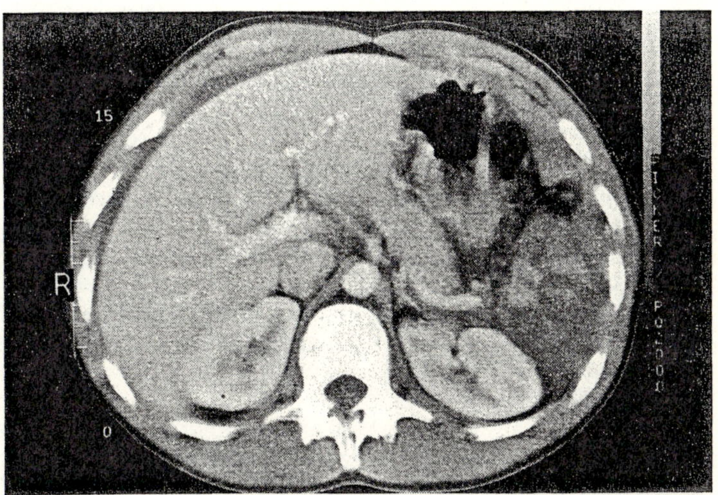

Fig. 4.1 Contrast-enhanced computed tomographic scan demonstrating complete disruption of the spleen. Some enhancing splenic tissue is seen anteriorly, but the majority of the spleen is devitalized, and therefore fails to take up contrast.

Questions

1. Detail the anatomical considerations relative to the assessment of a patient with blunt abdominal trauma.
2. Outline the principles of the clinical assessment of such patients.
3. Discuss the role of laboratory and radiological investigations as an adjunct to clinical assessment in these patients.
4. Describe the procedure of diagnostic peritoneal lavage (DPL) and its interpretation.
5. Classify splenic injuries and outline the principles of conservative therapy and splenic conservation at operation in the management of splenic trauma.
6. Discuss post-splenectomy sepsis.

Answers

1. When assessing a patient for specific injuries following trauma, the abdomen should be considered as four separate regions.
   (a) *Intrathoracic abdomen:*
      (i) Lies beneath the ribcage, inaccessible to palpation.
      (ii) Contains diaphragm, liver, spleen and stomach.
      (iii) Best investigated with DPL (also contrast-enhanced CT scan/ultrasound scan).
   (b) *Pelvic abdomen*
      (i) Lies in the hollow of the bony pelvis.
      (ii) Contains rectum, bladder, small intestine and female reproductive organs.
      (iii) Often there are few physical signs associated with injury.
      (iv) Investigated with cystourethrography/sigmoidoscopy, contrast-enhanced CT scan/ultrasound scan.
   (c) *Retroperitoneal abdomen*
      (i) Contains kidneys, ureters, pancreas, second and third parts of duodenum, aorta and vena cava.
      (ii) Physical examination and DPL are often unhelpful in diagnosis.
      (iii) Investigated with intravenous pyelography, CT scan (contrast-enhanced), ultrasound scan and angiography.

(d) *True abdomen*
  (i) Contains small and large intestines, distended bladder and gravid uterus.
  (ii) Injuries are usually associated with abdominal signs.

2. (a) *History.* An accurate history of the mechanism of injury aids in the management of blunt abdominal trauma. Collateral histories from witnesses or those in first attendance at the scene will help to determine the potential for injury. In road traffic accidents, the type of vehicle involved, the nature of any impact, the patient's position in the vehicle and whether a restraint device was being worn are all important factors. Information should also be obtained regarding the patient's level of consciousness at the scene and whether substance abuse is suspected. Finally, where possible, details of past medical history, medications and any known allergies should be obtained.

   (b) *Physical examination.* The initial assessment (primary survey) of the patient should follow the advanced trauma life support (ATLS) protocol, as defined by the Committee on Trauma of the American College of Surgeons (see Case 28). Having established the ABC of airway, breathing and circulation, the secondary survey consists of careful inspection of the patient, front and back, for ecchymoses and abrasions, which are pointers to intra-abdominal injury following blunt abdominal trauma. The respiratory pattern should be evaluated. Halted, laboured breathing may occur as a result of diaphragmatic irritation or upper abdominal injury, and may be a clue to significant abdominal trauma. Kehr's sign (shoulder pain on inspiration – present in the patient presented above) indicates diaphragmatic irritation from bleeding. Ribcage tenderness may indicate underlying rib fractures. There is a 20% chance of splenic injury and a 10% chance of hepatic injury with fractures of the left and right lower six ribs respectively.

   Abdominal signs are often absent initially, despite significant underlying injury, and repeated assessment of the abdomen in conjunction with careful monitoring of the vital signs is mandatory in order not to miss potentially life-threatening injuries. In a patient with continuing or refractory haemorrhagic shock which is unexplained, or in a patient who becomes unstable after an initial period of relative stability, early exploration of the abdomen is mandatory.

(c) *Abdominal examination: interpretation of physical findings.* Abdominal injury can involve:

(i) Vascular organs.
(ii) Solid organs.
(iii) Hollow organs.

Physical findings vary with the type of underlying injury present and the timing of onset of signs may be a function of the severity of the injury. As stated above, frequent re-examination is mandatory. Tenderness, particularly rebound tenderness, guarding or rigidity and absent bowel sounds are indicative of significant underlying peritoneal irritation. A pelvic fracture is suspected in the presence of suprapubic or lateral pelvic wall tenderness. The urinary meatus should be inspected for blood and the perineum for signs of injury. On rectal examination, anal sphincter tone, the position of the prostate and the integrity of the rectal wall are assessed.

3. (a) *Laboratory investigations.* The main function of haematological and biochemical investigations is for the establishment of baselines at the time of initial assessment, as subsequent changes may be the first sign of occult injury.

(i) Haematocrit reflects acute blood loss; serial measurement is helpful.
(ii) White cell count is non-specific.
(iii) Haemoglobin: fall is delayed.
(iv) Amylase: non-specific may be elevated without pancreatic trauma. It is often normal despite significant pancreatic injury, but elevated levels should raise suspicion.
(v) Urea/creatinine: baseline.
(vi) Electrolytes: baseline.
(vii) Glucose: baseline.
(viii) Coagulation screen: especially before blood transfusion.
(ix) Arterial blood gases in the unconscious or intubated patient.
(x) Urinalysis for detection of otherwise occult urological trauma.

(b) *Radiology.* Radiological procedures should only be performed under the strict supervision and monitoring of trained personnel, as the condition of a severely injured patient may change at any time. Such investigations may prove helpful where clinical assessment and laboratory investigations are inconclusive.

  (i) Chest X-ray for associated chest and diaphragmatic injuries; free air from perforated viscus; and bony injury.
  (ii) Abdominal X-ray for intraperitoneal haemorrhage; peritoneal contents 'floating' in ground-glass haze; retroperitoneal haemorrhage (loss of psoas/kidney shadow); duodenal injury (retroperitoneal stipling); and visceral perforation (free air).
  (iii) CT scan (contrast-enhanced).
  (iv) Ultrasound scan for solid organ injury.
  (v) Cystourethrography or intravenous pyelogram (IVP) for urological injury.
  (vi) Contrast duodenography for duodenial injury.
  (vii) Angiography for vascular injuries.
  (viii) Ultrasound or radionuclide scan as serial follow-up.

4. DPL can be utilized to detect significant intra-abdominal injury following blunt trauma. Positive lavage reduces delayed diagnosis and consequent morbidity and mortality. Negative lavage eliminates the need for unnecessary laparotomy.

   (a) *Indications*
      (i) Unconscious patient with signs of abdominal injury.
      (ii) Intoxicated patient with suspected abdominal injury.
      (iii) Multiply injured patient with unexplained shock.
      (iv) Injury suspected as a consequence of the mechanism of injury, but physical signs equivocal.
      (v) Spinal cord injury.
      (vi) Abdominal injury suspected; anaesthesia required for other injuries.

   (b) *Contraindications*
      (i) Obvious surgical abdomen – absolute.
      (ii) Previous abdominal surgery – relative.
      (iii) Pregnancy – relative.
      (iv) Morbid obesity – relative.

(c) *Procedures prior to DPL*
- (i) Pelvic radiograph: identify pelvic fractures.
- (ii) Gastric intubation + decompression.
- (iii) Bladder drainage.

(d) *Technique*
- (i) Periumbilical area shaved, prepped and draped with sterile towels.
- (ii) Area infiltrated with local anaesthetic.
- (iii) Incision to linea alba: rigorous haemostasis.
- (iv) Linea alba incised.
- (v) Peritoneum intubated with peritoneal dialysis catheter under direct vision.
  (*Semiopen technique:* Safe, quicker than open technique, avoids introduction of air.)
- (vi) Trocar withdrawn and catheter directed into pelvis.
- (vii) Initial aspirate for blood.
- (viii) Infusion of 1 l of warmed crystalloid solution.
- (ix) Lavage fluid syphoned from peritoneal cavity (container dropped to floor).
- (x) 75% effluent of lavage fluid required for valid procedure.

(e) *Interpretation*
- (i) $\geq$10 ml of frank blood aspirated – positive (tap).
- (ii) Faeces/bile aspirated – positive (tap).
- (iii) Lavage fluid is sent for laboratory analysis of red (RCC) and white cell (WCC) counts, amylase (LAM) and alkaline phosphatase (LAP) levels, and is tested for the presence of bile.
- (iv) RCC >100 000/mm^3 – positive.
- (v) RCC <20 000/mm^3 – negative.
- (vi) WCC >500/mm^3 – positive.
- (vii) LAM > 20 iu/l – positive.
- (viii) LAP $\geq$3 iu – positive.
- (ix) Bile detected in lavage fluid – positive.

5. Splenic injuries may be classified according to the extent and depth of trauma. Inspection of the spleen at laparotomy to determine the extent of injury is often not routine. However, in the majority of cases bleeding can be controlled while mobilization is completed, allowing assessment of the extent of trauma prior to embarking on splenectomy, without undue risk to the patient. In certain cases, conservation of the spleen may then be deemed feasible.

(a) *Classification of splenic injuries:*
   (i) Capsular tears may include small hilar vessels; there is no trauma to the underlying splenic pulp.
   (ii) Incomplete parenchymal tear does not approach the hilum.
   (iii) Extensive parenchymal tear extends up to hilum but does not divide it.
   (iv) Parenchymal tear involves complete division of the hilum, but with preservation of the blood supply to each fragment.
   (v) Fragmentation of the spleen with torn hilar vessels.
   (vi) Subcapsular haematoma (potential for delayed rupture).

(b) *Conservative management of splenic trauma:*
   (i) Patient haemodynamically stable on admission.
   (ii) Haemodynamic stability persists over the course of the first week in hospital, with no or modest transfusion requirements.
   (iii) No evidence of other intra-abdominal injuries.
   (iv) Equivocal or negative DPL.
   (v) Utilization of CT scanning, ultrasonography, radionuclide scanning or angiography, alone or in combination, for serial monitoring of splenic injury. Investigations should confirm superficial trauma of limited extent.
   (vi) Polyvalent pneumococcal vaccine should be administered before or immediately after splenectomy, with booster doses being given every 3 years.
   (vii) Prophylactic antibiotics should be continued for 2 years after surgery in the first instance. Thereafter antibiotics should always be administered before dental and other invasive procedures.
   (viii) Patients are advised of the increased risk of infection, and should carry an identity card to alert health care workers of their status.
   (ix) All infections should be treated as an emergency.

Further reading

Alexander RH and Procter HJ. (eds) *Advanced Trauma Life Support Course for Physicians, Student Manual.* American College of Surgeons, Chicago.

McAnena OJ, Moore EE and Marx JA. (1990) Initial evaluation of the patient with blunt abdominal trauma. *Surgical Clinics of North America* **70:** 495–515

McMahon MJ. (1988) Salvaging the spleen. *Surgery (Oxford)* **57:** 1348–1351
Moore EE, Mattox KL and Feliciano DV (eds) (1991) *Trauma.* Appleton & Lange, East Norwalk, Connecticut
Shackford SR and Moossa AR. (1988) Trauma. In: *Essential Surgical Practice,* Cushieri A, Giles GR, Moossa AR (eds). John Wright, Bristol

Terence J. Boyle
Oliver J. McAnena

Case 5 Macroscopic haematuria

A 63-year-old retired tobacconist was referred with a 2-month history of intermittent painless macroscopic haematuria. There were no associated symptoms. The patient had previously undergone coronary artery bypass grafting and was anticoagulated with warfarin. He had smoked 30 cigarettes a day until 5 years previously. On examination there was nothing to find apart from a moderately enlarged benign-feeling prostate gland. Dipstick analysis of normal-looking urine was positive for blood.

Questions

1. What is the differential diagnosis of macroscopic haematuria?
2. What are the important factors on history and examination which may help pinpoint the cause for haematuria?
3. How would you investigate macroscopic haematuria?

Answers

1. Macroscopic haematuria is a significant symptom that warrants urgent investigation as approximately 20% of these patients have a neoplasm of the urinary tract. Macroscopic haematuria may be caused by a large number of diseases, some of which are frequently encountered, whilst others are uncommon (Table 5.1). The causes of macroscopic haematuria may also be classified according to the site of bleeding, under the headings of glomerular and non-glomerular (urological) bleeding.
2. In a patient presenting with macroscopic haematuria pain, frequency, urgency, dysuria and symptoms of outflow obstruction may help indicate the underlying cause. Painless macroscopic haematuria is taken to indicate a neoplasm of the urinary tract until proven otherwise. Pain, especially colic, may indicate a urinary tract stone but passage of clots from a bleeding renal cell carcinoma or upper tract tumour may also produce colic (clot colic). A dull loin ache may be

Table 5.1 Common and uncommon causes of haematuria

Common causes
Transitional cell carcinoma
Renal cell carcinoma
Urinary tract infection
Urolithiasis
Sickle-cell disease
Schistosomiasis
Glomerulonephritis
Trauma
Benign prostatic hyperplasia
Prostatic adenocarcinoma
Uncommon causes
Blood dyscrasias
Polycystic kidney
Horseshoe kidney
Medullary sponge kidney
Renal artery stenosis
Haemangioma
Systemic lupus erythematosus
Post-exercise haematuria

caused by obstruction from an upper tract tumour or a large renal pelvis stone. Frequency, urgency and dysuria in association with haematuria may indicate infective cystitis. However, these symptoms in a man may occasionally be due to carcinoma-*in-situ*. Associated fevers suggest pyelonephritis. In older men, symptoms of bladder outflow obstruction indicate a benign or malignant enlargement of the prostate gland, both of which may cause macroscopic haematuria.

Past medical history and medications are also relevant. Patients on anticoagulants may have haematuria if poorly controlled. Patients with a history of easy bruising and bleeding problems after dental extractions or minor surgery may have blood dyscrasis. A past history of glomerulonephritis may indicate a glomerular cause, whilst a history of ingestion of large amounts of analgesics may suggest increased risk of papillary necrosis which may cause haematuria. Occasionally, fit young adults may describe painless macroscopic haematuria after vigorous exercise, which is a well-recognized entity entitled post-exercise haematuria. A family history of renal disease may point to an inherited disease such as Alport's syndrome or polycystic kidneys.

The presence of clots and the timing of the bleeding may also be important. Bleeding at the start of micturition may indicate a lesion in the urethra distal to the external sphincter, whilst bleeding at the end of micturition may indicate pathology in the region of the bladder neck. Bleeding throughout the urinary stream indicates a source in the bladder, kidney or upper tracts.

Physical examination should include inspection for anaemia, hypertension, jaundice and the systemic effects of advanced malignant disease. Abdominal examination may reveal a renal mass due to tumour, hydronephrosis or polycystic kidneys. Renal angle tenderness implies inflammation. A palpable bladder indicates significant outflow obstruction. Rectal examination of the prostate to distinguish malignant and benign enlargement is important. However, a majority of patients with macroscopic haematuria have no obvious abnormalities on physical examination.

3. (a) *Urinalysis.* A dipstick test detects intact red blood cells, free haemoglobin and myoglobin. However, oxidizing agents such as hypochlorite may lead to false-positive reactions, whilst large amounts of reducing agents such as vitamin C may cause false-negative results. Thus, haematuria detected by dipstick testing should be confirmed by urine microscopy. A freshly voided overnight sample is ideal. The urine specimen is centrifuged and the sediment is examined at low and high power. The presence of three or fewer erythrocytes per high-powered field is accepted by most authorities as normal. Approximately 3% of normal individuals will have more than three erythrocytes per high-powered field. In addition to testing for erythrocytes, the urine is examined for white blood cells, protein, casts and bacteria. The presence of proteinuria and casts suggests a glomerular origin. A raised urinary white cell count, especially in the presence of bacteria, suggests an infective cause. An increased number of urinary white blood cells may also occur with calculi or tumours. Persistent sterile pyuria should raise suspicions of tuberculosis.

   Red blood cell morphology may be used to help pinpoint the source of bleeding. Red blood cells from glomerular and tubulointerstitial disease are frequently distorted (dysmorphic), whilst red blood cells from non-glomerular lesions are usually isomorphic. Phase-contrast microscopy may be used to study red blood cell morphology. Alternatively, Coulter counter analysis of mean corpuscular diameters may distinguish between dysmorphic and isomorphic red blood cells. These latter investigations are usually reserved for patients with persistent haematuria in whom standard investigations have failed to demonstrate a cause. However, in the presence of proteinuria and/or urinary casts, these investigations should be used early in the course of the investigation to help decide whether renal or urological work-up is more appropriate.

Urine may also be sent for cytological examination, especially where risk factors for transitional cell carcinoma such as smoking or occupational exposure to aromatic amines exists. Urine cytology is particularly sensitive for high-grade tumours but less so for low-grade tumours, so that a negative result is not conclusive.

(b) *Haematological investigations.* A full blood count, erythrocyte sedimentation rate (ESR) and serum creatinine, urea and electrolytes are worthwhile investigations which may demonstrate anaemia, polycythaemia, abnormal ESR or renal impairment. In young black men sickle-cell disease or trait may account for up to one-third of cases of haematuria and should be routinely tested for.

(c) *Radiological investigation.* An intravenous urogram (IVU) is the standard investigation unless there is an allergy to contrast, in which case an ultrasound and plain abdominal film may be used. Distortion of the collecting system may be due to a renal cell carcinoma, reflux nephropathy, calculi, sloughed renal papilla or caliceal tumour. Upper tract tumours may cause a filling defect in the renal pelvis or ureter, as may non-opaque calculi. Apparent filling defects may sometimes be caused by overlying bowel gas or compression by a vessel. Patients with a filling defect on IVU should have a retrograde ureterogram at the time of cystoscopy. Patients with distortion of the collecting system and a suspected renal tumour should have a renal ultrasound with particular attention to the renal vein and inferior vena cava to rule out tumour thrombus. Computed tomography (CT) and magnetic resonance imaging (MRI) are not used as first-line investigations but may have a role to play in staging tumours prior to surgery.

(d) *Cystoscopy.* A thorough examination of the urethra and bladder can be achieved using a flexible cystoscope. Flexible cystoscopy can be performed on an outpatient basis using local anaesthetic jelly or lubrication alone. Where there is a suspected filling defect on IVU, rigid cystoscopy under general anaesthesia with retrograde ureterography is indicated. The ureteral catheter can also be used to obtain saline washings from the suspicious area for cytological examination. In the occasional case where a combination of retrograde ureterography and cytology fails to resolve the nature of a filling defect, a flexible ureterorenoscope may be used to visualize and biopsy the suspicious area.

(e) *Angiography.* Radionuclide angiography or contrast arteriography may help confirm and localize an arteriovenous fistula, which is an uncommon cause of haematuria seen after renal needle biopsy, trauma or partial nephrectomy.

To summarize, macroscopic haematuria is a significant symptom that indicates a neoplasm of the genitourinary tract in up to 20% of cases. In most cases a cause can be demonstrated. In the absence of a demonstrable cause for haematuria, the patient should be reassured but advised to return for further assessment if the haematuria recurs or new symptoms develop.

Andrew McEvoy
Tom Creagh

Case 6 Appendix mass

You are travelling incognito on a cargo ship with 11 other passengers. In mid Pacific Ocean, a 28-year-old crew member has been ill with abdominal pain for 5 days, when the captain discovers that you are a trainee surgeon, so you are asked to go and see the seaman professionally.

The patient says that he has previously been very fit, until 5 days ago, when he developed central abdominal pain which moved to the right iliac fossa, where it has remained as a steady severe ache. He has vomited once or twice and his bowels have worked twice without diarrhoea. The sickbay attendant has been giving him a combination of co-proxamol, gin and ampicillin, which seems to have made things bearable. Over the last day, the pain has been marginally better rather than worse. He is considerably thirsty. There are no urinary symptoms and no relevant past history.

On examination, the patient looks flushed and unwell: temperature 38°C, pulse 100 beats/min. The chest and heart are normal. The tongue is furred with a foetor. The abdomen is generally tender, but not grossly so, and there is a 10-cm tender mass in the right iliac fossa arising out of the pelvis. Rectal examination is normal.

Questions

1. What should you do?
   (a) Radio and divert the ship to the nearest large port?
   (b) Radio, take advice and manage the case conservatively – if so, how?
   (c) Radio, sort out the ship's emergency operating kit and proceed to operate under spinal anaestheisa (in which you happen to be proficient)?
2. How would you manage things differently, if this patient turned up at your previous UK hospital with the same history and clinical findings?

Answers

1. (a) Your patient does not have generalized peritonitis. The most likely diagnosis is appendix mass, which means a phlegmon of adherent omentum and small bowel or a locally inflamed, possibly locally perforated, appendicitis. At present, the body seems to be winning against the infective process.

   Immediate operation is contraindicated – you are likely to make things worse.

   Symptomatic treatment is indicated – do not divert the ship!

   (b) Yes, of course you should use the radio. The advice you receive should be to manage the case conservatively, but what does this mean?

   First, you need to initiate appropriate antibiotic therapy against the bacteria which are likely to be involved – this means against the aerobes and anaerobes. So far, your patient has had inappropriate antibiotic therapy (ampicillin), which will only affect the aerobic organisms (coliforms, etc.). Numerous trials have shown that this is an ineffective form of treatment. You must cover the anaerobic bacteria (e.g. *Bacteroides*) as well. Metronidazole suppositories three times a day would be satisfactory in addition to the oral ampicillin.

   Hydration needs to be secured. If your patient is under-hydrated (and he says he is thirsty), then he needs an intravenous infusion as well, giving 3 l/day. Your ship's medical stores should be able to run to this.

   Now take a skin pencil (magic marker will do) and mark the size of the mass. Redraw your line each day and observe progress. If the mass gets smaller, that is fine. If the mass stays static, this is acceptable. If the mass enlarges, divert the ship!

   (c) Immediate operation is a disastrous idea at this stage – many acute operations by inexperienced surgeons at this stage of an appendix mass end up in a right hemicolectomy or worse. You cannot do a right hemicolectomy with inadequate anaestheisa, possibly at all, and certainly not on your own at sea! The most you should contemplate would be a right iliac fossa incicion under local anaesthesia, which might allow you to drain the appendix abscess and this could be life-saving.

2. In your usual hospital, I would expect you to proceed more or less in the same manner as in (b), albeit with more tests.

   You need to understand that during the past 5 days, the body has fought the inflamed appendix to a standstill and we now need to see whether, with a little help from antibiotics, the condition will quietly resolve, leaving a scarred fibrous appendix, or whether the infective process is going to win and lead to an increasing pelvic abscess, septicaemia and death (in which case you do need to intervene).

   So, put up a drip, measure full blood count, urea and electrolytes, take a plain abdominal X-ray and ultrasound scan, start metronidazole plus ampicillin or gentamicin and await developments.

   Serial clinical observation will show that 80–90% of patients quickly get better. The pain disappears, the mass starts to reduce in size and eventually resolves and the patient goes home, still with a palpable mass, that is by now non-tender and painless. In 10–20% of patients the mass gets larger, or the patient becomes toxic. In this situation, senior help is needed and although in theory simple drainage of the abscess either under screened radiological control or at open operation sounds a good idea, most operations, in my experience, end up with some form of limited right hemicolectomy (see review cited below).

   (a) *Further investigation.* In patients older than your 28-year-old seaman (e.g. those over perhaps 40 years of age), interval tests need to be performed in the outpatient clinic to exclude an underlying caecal tumour. Thus the patient must undergo either a barium enema or colonoscopy or both. In a previously fit man of 28, such as your patient, I believe that such tests are unnecessary.

       You must make certain that the mass disappears *completely*, and remains absent thereafter.

   (b) *Outcome.* In the 80–90% of patients with appendix mass who have been treated conservatively, conventional wisdom dictates that an interval appendicectomy is performed at 3 months, to remove the risk of a second episode of severe appendicitis. Scientific validation for this course of action is considerably scanty, yet most surgeons of my acquaintance do believe this is the right thing to do.

       In the recent review cited under Further reading below, the authors come down on the side of not doing an interval appendicectomy, but admit that the evidence for this view is also lacking! If you proposed to argue this approach in an examination, you had better read the review itself with some care.

In the 10–20% who get worse rather than better with conservative treatment, the situation is resolved for you by some form of emergency operation. A small proportion of these patients will eventually proceed to multiple complications and eventual death.

(c) *Late complications.* A minority – perhaps 10% – of patients coming from both the conservatively managed group and the operatively managed group, will later develop episodes of adhesive obstruction, which will require management in its own right.

Further reading

Nitecki S, Assalia A and Schein M. (1993) Contemporary management of the appendiceal mass. *British Journal of Surgery* **80:** 18–20

M.J. Kelly

Case 7 Deep vein thrombosis and pulmonary embolism

An obese 50-year-old woman was admitted for radical surgical treatment of a stage IIb ovarian carcinoma. Graduated compression thromboembolic deterrent stockings (TEDS) were used for deep vein thrombosis (DVT) prophylaxis. Following extensive surgery, the patient remained in bed for 3 days. On the fifth postoperative day she complained of a mild ache in the groin but there were no clinical signs of venous obstruction; Doppler examination of the femoral vein was normal. Ten days after surgery the patient collapsed in the bathroom. She was hypotensive with a respiratory rate of 40 breaths/min. Her oxygen saturation was 68% measured by pulse oximetry and a chest X-ray, electrocardiogram (ECG) and blood gases all supported a provisional diagnosis of pulmonary embolism (PE).

Questions

1. What predisposing factors for DVT and PE did this patient have?
2. How should a possible DVT have been diagnosed or excluded on day 5?
3. What are the clinical features of PE and how would you investigate and manage the patient on day 10?
4. What is the relationship between DVT and PE, and its implications for management?
5. Discuss DVT prophylaxis for the various categories of patient. Do you agree with the prophylaxis in this case?

Answers

1. The predisposing factors for venous thromboembolism are: changes in blood flow, changes in the vessel wall and changes in blood-clotting activity (Virchow's triad). The reduction in blood flow occurs as a consequence of immobilization and absence of calf muscle contraction; this leads to

venous stasis, local hypoxia and an increase in coagulability. Local hypoxia in valve pockets causes vein wall damage, as does any form of direct trauma to the veins, e.g. in pelvic surgery or during total hip replacement. Initiation of the clotting cascade follows and a thrombus develops. Alterations in blood coagulability are seen in patients with deficiency of natural anticoagulants (e.g. antithrombin III, protein C, protein S), women with high oestrogen levels (pregnancy, oral contraceptives) and in many patients with malignancy. Increasing age is also a risk factor and all patients over 40 years of age have an increased risk. This patient had a number of risk factors for DVT, with the overall risk being determined by the product of the individual risk factors rather than the simple additive sum. The risk factors in this case include obesity, age and sex, pelvic surgery, the presence of cancer and prolonged immobilization.

2. Clinical diagnosis of DVT is notoriously inaccurate. It is wrong in 50% of cases and is neither sensitive nor specific. DVT is asymptomatic in many patients because of incomplete occlusion of the vein lumen by the thrombus, particularly in large proximal veins. Anatomical anomalies with thrombosis of only one vein of a duplicated system may also be present. Moreover, superficial collateral circulation and stasis with oedema distally do not occur following a DVT. Thus, many DVTs are silent.

   Venography remains the gold standard in the diagnosis of DVT. Venous Doppler assessment (sound only) and duplex scanning (sound and vision) are increasingly being used in the diagnosis of DVT. Diagnosing a proximal DVT with Doppler alone is often inaccurate as incomplete occlusion of the vein fails to produce the characteristic loss of flow augmentation and absence of phasic flow with respiration. Duplex scanning is far more accurate; vein compressibility and partial occlusion of the vein can be seen and flow changes detected. Inaccuracies with non-occluding iliac vein thrombosis may occur as visualization in the pelvis is difficult. This is a problem with venography in this area also. Duplex scanning performed by a skilled technician is the preferred venous imaging technique in many centres today.

   On day 5 postoperatively, this patient had local symptoms consistent with an acute non-occluding thrombosis in the femoral vein. Because of the patient's obvious increased risk of developing a DVT, treatment by anticoagulation should have been instituted until the diagnosis was excluded by either venography or duplex scanning. Standard treatment for DVT is immediate heparinization in the form of a bolus dose followed by a continuous heparin infusion. The activated partial thromboplastin time (APTT) should be in a range of 1.5–2.5 times the control. For long-term anticoagulation warfarin is required for 3–6 months. Warfarin is usually started as soon as the diagnosis of DVT is confirmed, a loading dose is given usually in divided doses and once the prothrombin time (PT) reaches 2–2½ times the control value, a maintenance dose is given. During the early stages of warfarin therapy a hypercoagulable state may exist before vitamin K-dependent factors with longer half-lives (II, IX, X) are sufficiently inhibited. Hence, heparin therapy should continue for 5 days after the start of warfarin, even though the international normalized ratio (INR) may reflect a therapeutic warfarin effect after 2–3 days.

Thrombolytic therapy with streptokinase or tissue plasminogen activator may have a limited role in those cases of complete occlusion of the femoral or iliac vein causing a grossly swollen limb. This treatment requires skilled interventional radiology to place the catheter within the clot, and although it produces more rapid relief of the occlusive symptoms, it has not been shown to reduce the incidence of long-term chronic venous problems.

3. The diagnosis of pulmonary embolism is made on the clinical evidence and confirmed by a number of investigations. The clinical signs associated with a PE depend on the size of the embolus and the cardiopulmonary status of the patient. They range from chest pain, acute breathlessness and haemoptysis to varying degrees of collapse, including sudden death. A chest radiograph excludes other causes of acute breathlessness but rarely are obvious changes in the pulmonary markings seen initially in a patient with a PE. Similarly, an ECG excludes a myocardial infarct but the classical changes of S-wave depression in lead 1 and Q- and T-wave changes in lead 3 are rare. Hypoxia and hypocarbia on arterial blood-gas analysis provide non-specific supportive evidence for a diagnosis of PE. Ventilation–perfusion isotope scans produce a definite diagnosis in less than 50% of cases. Pulmonary arteriography is the best method for

confirming the diagnosis of PE, but it is invasive and dangerous in the high-risk patient and is rarely performed outside specialist centres.

The management of PE includes general supportive measures such as administration of oxygen and haemodynamic support if there has been significant right ventricular strain. Specific treatment of the thromboembolic process using heparin and warfarin is similar to that for a DVT except that heparin is given for up to 1 week and warfarin for up to 1 year. Thrombolytic therapy may accelerate resolution of emboli and improve cardiopulmonary status, particularly where cardiac output is compromised. Pulmonary embolectomy is rarely attempted now. Inferior vena caval filters are usually considered for recurrent pulmonary emboli despite adequate anticoagulation, inability to tolerate anticoagulatoin, a large free-floating thrombus in the ileofemoral vein and following pulmonary embolectomy.

4. Pulmonary emboli are found at autopsy in about one-third of patients dying in hospital. The majority of fatal pulmonary emboli occur in patients over 50 years of age, with a peak at around 70 years. The relationship between PE and lower limb DVT is controversial. About 15–20% of thrombi in the legs embolize. Thrombi usually originate in the calf veins and propagate proximally to the larger veins above the knee. Pulmonary emboli usually arise from the thrombi in the large veins proximal to the knee, but rarely from isolated thrombi in the calf veins. Thrombi will also arise *de novo* in the large proximal veins if they have been directly injured – as in hip surgery – and these obviously have a high potential to embolize.

   All above-knee DVTs should be treated. However, controversy exists as to whether all calf DVTs should be treated. The majority of patients with calf vein DVT do not develop proximal extension and complications rarely occur in this group. It is recommended that serial follow-up with duplex scans and selective therapy to patients with propagation is the most appropriate management. This limits the risks and costs of anticoagulation, particularly in the elderly who would benefit most.

5. Prophylaxis is one of the most important aspects of the management of DVT. Prophylaxis should be initiated before surgery and should be continued until the patient is no longer exposed to the various risk factors already discussed.

Mechanical prophylaxis aims to increase venous flow and minimize the risk of thrombosis secondary to stasis. Graduated elastic compression stockings increase the velocity of venous blood flow from the legs and decrease the incidence of DVT by 50% when used alone. External pneumatic compression devices applied to the legs or foot increase venous return by simulating the effect of walking. Sequential compression of the veins has also been shown to have the additional effect of increasing fibrinolytic activity within the blood. These devices are recommended for patients where anticoagulation is contraindicated, such as in those undergoing neurosurgical procedures and in those with haemorrhagic strokes. They are also used in conjunction with pharmacological agents as they appear to have additive effects in keeping the risk of thrombosis to a minimum.

Low-dose heparin is the most popular method of pharmacological prophylaxis. The secondary benefit of producing a large reduction in PE has also been documented since the introduction of DVT prophylaxis. However, a direct correlation between prophylaxis and PE has not been shown as the latter is often diagnosed clinically without a postmortem. All circumstantial evidence shows a relationship. Low-dose heparin is used in all patients over the age of 40 undergoing an operation lasting longer than 30 min.

Low-molecular-weight heparin is said to increase the antithrombotic activity of heparin without increasing the risk of haemorrhagic complications. It is proving more effective than low-dose heparin in high-risk orthopaedic patients. Its superiority over standard low-dose heparin in elderly patients with malignancy is also likely, although not yet proven. It has the shared advantage with low-dose heparin of not requiring monitoring.

Intravenous dextran is also effective but requires a continuous intravenous infusion and carries the risk of fluid overload and allergic reactions. It also interferes with subsequent cross-matching of blood.

Adjusted-dose warfarin is also used in high-risk orthopaedic patients and is highly effective. Haemorrhagic complications and the need for continuous monitoring have restricted its use.

In our patient we would have used low-dose heparin in conjunction with TED stockings and intermittent pneumatic compression devices used during surgery.

Further reading

Bergqvist D, Comerota AJ, Nicolaides AN and Scurr JH. (1994) *Prevention of Venous Thromboembolism*. Med-Orion, London

Greenfield LJ. (1993) Venous thrombosis and pulmonary thromboembolism. In: *Surgery, Scientific Principles and Practice*, Mulholland M, Oldham KT, Zelenock GB (eds). JP Lippincott, Philadelphia

Paul Burke
Irwin Mohan

Case 8 Pyloric stenosis

A 63-year-old male presented to his local hospital complaining of increasing central abdominal pain and vomiting. This had started 2 weeks previously but had become more severe over the last 2 days. Initially the symptoms had been relieved by antacids but now he gained no relief from these medications. He had continued trying to eat and drink but felt bloated and this was relieved when he vomited. The vomiting had been profuse. He had noticed that his urine was dark and that he was not passing urine very often. He felt thirsty.

On examination he was a thin man who appeared malnourished. He was drawn and had a dry tongue. His pulse and blood pressure were unremarkable but his jugular venous pressure could only be seen when lying down and was obviously low. His abdomen was distended and he was tender in his epigastrium. A succession splash could be elicited.

Investigations revealed a mild anaemia with a haemoglobin of 10.4 g/dl; white blood cells 10.0×10^9/l and platelets 303. His electrolytes were Na 136, K 3.3, Cl 83, urea 17.8 mmol and creatinine 210 μmol/l. Arterial blood-gas analysis showed pH 7.54; $Paco_2$ 5.1 kPa; Pao_2 12 kPa. His bicarbonate was 37 mmol/l.

Questions

1. What is the likely diagnosis?
2. What treatment should be initiated and why?
3. Are there any further investigations you would like?
4. What is the pathophysiological basis of the metabolic disturbance?

Answers

1. The diagnosis is pyloric stenosis with the probable underlying cause due to a duodenal ulcer. The triad of complaints of upper abdominal fullness, nausea and vomiting is usually present. Pain is not a consistent feature but a past history of indigestion, often over a long period of time, may be elicited. The patient's main concern may be the abdominal pain; antacids initially helped but now give him no relief. The pain

may however be relieved by vomiting; this occasionally contains recognizable material from meals eaten days before.

2. The assessment and treatment of this condition require understanding of the problems presenting. These are dehydration, metabolic alkalosis due to acid loss and then the physical mechanism which has caused it. The first disturbances involves volume depletion and the loss of H^+Cl^- from the stomach consequent to the vomiting. Attempts by parietal cells to maintain hydrogen ion production also produce HCO_3^-.

   Initial assessment of the fluid status of the patient is important. Although his cardiovascular parameters appear normal, the raised urea and creatinine are a cause for concern and probably indicate a prolonged period of effective dehydration. He has lost water. It is likely that to see renal changes there must be at least a 10–20% intravascular deficit. the absence of cardiovascular changes is a consequence of this dehydration occurring slowly and his ability to compensate effectively. In a compensated patient an acidosis from hypoperfusion is unlikely to develop until the perfusion problem is profound and in this case would be masked by the metabolic alkalosis, which will be described below. Expansion of his intravascular compartment is both necessary and urgent. It is immaterial whether colloids or crystalloids are used but a smaller volume of colloid, than saline, will achieve expansion of the intravascular compartment. A volume in the order of 10% of his estimated blood volume should be given in the first instance. (Rule of thumb: blood volume is about 100 ml/kg.) A change in blood pressure and pulse may sometimes be seen as the pressure, while within normal limits, may be lower than the patient's normal value.

   The metabolic problem that this patient demonstrates is hydrogen ion loss in association with chloride loss from the stomach. The concentration of Cl in the vomitus is 100 mmol/l, Na 45 mmol/l and K 10 mmol/l. There is increased production of bicarbonate to try and replace the hydrogen ions.

$$H_2O + CO_2 = H_2CO_3 = H^+ + HCO_3^-$$

   Increased levels of bicarbonate in the blood exceed the renal threshold at approximately 28 mmol/l, and at this point the anion is lost into the urine, taking with it an obligatory cation. With a marked hydrogen ion deficit the kidney excretes either potassium or sodium preferentially to conserve hydrogen. The kidney is hampered however by the fact that sodium is absorbed passively along with chloride in the proximal tubule. Since there is a deficiency of chloride, more sodium is available in the distal tubule and is absorbed preferentially in exchange for K^+. The problem is compounded by dehydration in two ways. First, dehydration triggers aldosterone release and conservation of sodium and water with increased potassium loss, and second, the low glomerular filtration rate results in reduced renal bicarbonate excretion. This is part of the cause of the potassium loss; the rest moves intracellularly again compensating for intracellular accumulation of HCO_3^-.

The keystones of treatment are intravasuclar repletion followed by replacement of the salt and water loss from the extracellular space. Saline solutions containing sodium and chloride will, when intravascularly replete, allow rehydration of the extracellular space. As renal function returns with a normal glomerular filtration rate the kidneys will start correcting the alkalosis. The potassium deficit will become overt and so aggressive potassium replacement should commence with the saline infusion. The plasma bicarbonate value, while indicating alkalosis, should also indicate potassium deficiency.

It is worth comment that the increase in bicarbonate, alkalosis, which occurs should, in theory, be compensated for by an increase in the $Paco_2$. The respiratory centre is not sensitive to alkalosis and it is unusual for the carbon dioxide to be increased in these patients unless there is underlying respiratory disease. Since there is no compensatory increase in $Paco_2$, there is an increase in extracellular pH.

In the meantime the stomach should be decompressed with a nasogastric tube and the patient should be given nil by mouth. Drug treatment with H_2-antagonists or omeprazole is also helpful as many cases have ongoing duodenal ulceration.

3. Plain abdominal X-rays may show a large gastric fluid level but a barium examination should wait until the stomach has been emptied, otherwise little information will be obtained. Gastroscopy is invaluable and may help to exclude a possible obstructive neoplasm.
4. When these meaures are complete, investigation of the underlying cause can commence and definitive treatment

can be instituted. Surgery is the most effective treatment in any patient who fails to settle completely within a week of starting treatment, even for those who are able to take liquids successfully. The surgical options are vagotomy and gastric resection, vagotomy and pyloroplasty and intra-operative dilation with vagotomy. Recent interest has reported the success of endoscopic balloon dilatation, with a sustained response to follow-up of 2.5 years in up to two-thirds of patients treated.

Further reading

Oh M and Carroll H. (1992) Disorders of sodium metabolism: hypernatraemia and hyponatraemia. *Critical Care Medicine* **9:** 630–632

Cohen R. (1991) Roles of the liver and kidney in acid–base regulation and its disorders. *British Journal of Anaesthesia* **67:** 154–164

Hawker R. (1982) *Notebook of Medical Physiology, Renal and body Fluids.* Churchill Livingstone, Edinburgh

Mayne P. (1994) *Clinical Chemistry in Diagnosis and Treatment,* 6th edn. Edward Arnold, London

Neil Soni
Geoffrey Raine

Case 9 Head injury and transport of critically ill patients

A young adult male has been found unconscious beside his bicycle in a remote area of the country. He has been admitted to the local hospital and, assuming that he has sustained a head injury, his doctors have contacted the regional neurosurgical centre with a request to transfer him for ongoing management.

Questions

1. What initial management should be provided and what possible causes should be excluded?
2. What are the indications and contraindications for transfer?
3. Describe what should be done before transfer.
4. How should the transfer be undertaken?
5. What steps should the receiving centre make to prepare for his arrival?

Answers

1. The initial management should consist of resuscitation according to Advanced Trauma Life Support (ATLS) protocols. The commonest cause of death following a head injury occurs in the first 10 min from airway obstruction. The airway should be secured and intermittent positive-pressure ventilation instituted if spontaneous respiration is depressed. Intubation should then be undertaken at the earliest opportunity, and unless there is no response to painful stimuli, an induction agent and muscle relaxant must be used.

   A large-bore cannula must be inserted and a fluid challenge administered if there is hypotension.

   The neck must be assumed to be unstable, and fully immobilized. The minimum monitoring is an electrocardiogram, pulse oximeter and non-invasive blood pressure. The patient should be examined for other injuries.

   Non-neurological causes include hypo- and hyperglycaemia, drug overdose and myocardial pathology. The possibility of a bleed from a cerebral aneurysm or arteriovenous malformation should not be overlooked. A careful examination of the patient's pockets for drugs or medical alerts should be undertaken. The blood sugar should be measured and blood and urine sent for drug screening.

2. The indications for transfer to a neurosurgical centre are for surgical intervention for an extradural or subdural haematoma. A computed tomography (CT) scan is thus a prerequisite. Up to one-third of transfers are necessary because of the lack of scanning facilities locally. Transfer may also be necessary if there are no free intensive care beds in the receiving hospital.

   Interhospital transfer should only be undertaken following adequate resuscitation when the patient is stable. The patient can only be safely transferred with an adequate standard of accompanying staff and monitoring equipment.

3. Unless transfer needs to be undertaken immediately, the patient should be transferred to intensive care. An arterial catheter should be inserted and ventilation undertaken to achieve a $P\text{CO}_2$ of 3.5 kPa. A multilumen central catheter and urinary catheter should also be inserted. Sedation should be given so that there is no rise in pulse or blood pressure with nursing or surgical procedures. Drugs used for this purpose include propofol, benzodiazepines and narcotics. Patients may need preloading with fluids to avoid hypotension. The blood pressure should not be allowed to fall, and if hypotension does not respond to a fluid challenge, the early use of inotropes should be considered.

   A non-depolarizing muscle relaxant should be used to avoid any coughing or gagging on ventilation and suction.

   Blood should be cross-matched, and tetanus toxoid given if appropriate. Nimodipine may help prevent vascular spasm but is more commonly used for cerebral aneurysms. The use of steroids and osmotic diuretics is uncommon as they have not been proved to be beneficial.

   Other treatment may include insertion of an intracranial pressure monitor or the use of a cerebral function monitor. The patient should be kept normothermic, especially if interhospital transfer is planned, and the use of convective warming devices and fluid warmers is to be recommended.

4. Interhospital transfer should be the decision of the sending hospital consultant following discussion with an acceptance

of the patient by the receiving hospital consultant. The transferring doctor should undertake the transfer on this basis unless he or she considers that it is unsafe.

The three considerations are the vehicle, the team and the equipment. Minimum standards have been set down and published.

Short-distance transfers of less than 50 km (about 30 miles) and within a single conurbation are best undertaken by road ambulance. Most commonly, the only vehicle available will be a front-line ambulance from the local ambulance service. Ideally, the trolley should be mounted to facilitate all-round access, the monitoring equipment must be able to be securely fastened in view of the team, and the team must be seated and restrained. The doctor should be at the head of the patient.

Longer-distance transfers are best undertaken by helicopter. The helicopter reduces the amount of vibration, vertical buffeting and accelerational forces, all of which have been shown to be deleterious to a head-injured patient and to result in a rise in intracranial pressure, a fall in blood pressure and an increase in pulmonary shunting. The helicopter tips nose-down to accelerate and nose-up to brake, so a patient loaded longitudinally will compensate for these forces. A helicopter, as a result, may reduce mortality by up to a half compared with land-based transfers, as well as reduce the transit time during which the patient is at risk.

The minimum team consists of a doctor and nurse. Both should be of adequate seniority and from a relevant specialty. They should be properly clothed and not have any other responsibilities during or immediately after the estimated time of return. If a helicopter is to be used, they must have received specific training in care of the patient in the air as well as emergency drills. In practice this makes the use of a proper transfer service mandatory.

The minimum amount of monitoring is:

(a) Electrocardiogram.
(b) Pulse oximetry.
(c) Blood pressure measurement.
(d) Positive-pressure ventilation.
(e) Defibrillator.
(f) Oxygen.
(g) Suction.

(h) Facilities for endotracheal intubation.
(i) Intravenous fluid administration.
(j) Appropriate drugs for resuscitation.

All the monitors must be battery-powered and there must be sufficient power for bedside-to-bedside monitoring as well as unexpected delays. Equally there must be ample oxygen, and it cannot be assumed that the ambulance supply will have compatible connectors.

The patient must be set up for transfer in the hospital. All monitors must be moved across and lines adequately secured. Limbs must be padded to prevent pressure area problems or trauma. Monitors must not be placed on the patient. Adequate thermal insulation must be in hand.

The transferring team must receive a formal handover, as well as notes, X-rays and any blood. The relatives must be informed, told of the potential risk and prevented from chasing the ambulance. The decision for them to travel in the ambulance is that of the team leader. The relatives must then be provided with transport and directions.

In transit, the need for resuscitation or other interventions should be rare, and normally indicates inadequate pre-transfer stabilization. A proper record should be kept of relevant parameters. The transfer should not be undertaken at high speed and accelerational forces should be minimized.

5. The receiving hospital should have told the team where to take the patient in the hospital, and adequate facilities should be present at that site to deal with in-transit complications, the need to take over monitoring or ventilation urgently and to assess the patient. There should once again be a formal handover to a named doctor.

   The transfer team should have facilities for rest and refreshments and telephone facilities to contact their hospital. Follow-up of the patient following transfer should be encouraged.

Further reading

Bristow A *et al.* (1991) Medical helicopter systems – recommended minimum standards for patient management. *Journal of the Royal Society of Medicine* **84:** 242–244

Aubrey Bristow

Case 10 Organ donation

A 35-year-old man with insulin-dependent diabetes and a previously undiagnosed primary cerebral lesion is admitted to the intensive care unit in deep coma.

Following a period of examination and investigation, a diagnosis of brainstem death is suspected.

The first set of brainstem death tests has been completed and each individual test failed to initiate any response. Final confirmatory testing is planned in a few hours.

Clinical picture

The patient is ventilated on intermittent positive pressure.

Ventilation	$Fi\text{O}_2$	35% O_2
Arterial blood gases	$Pa\text{O}_2$	15 kPa
	$Pa\text{CO}_2$	4.7 kPa
	pH	7.38
	Base excess	−1 mmol/l
Haematology	White cell count	6.3×10^9/l
	Haemoglobin	11 g/dl
	Platelets	290×10^9
Biochemistry	Na	143 mmol/l
	K	4.0 mmol/l
	Urea	17 mmol/l
	Creatinine	92 μmol/l
	Alanine aminotransferase (ALT)	30 iu/l
	Aspartate aminotransferase (AST)	32 iu/l
	Alkaline phosphatase	180 iu/l
	Bilirubin	8 μmol/l
	Albumin	30 g/l

Questions

1. Would this patient be suitable for organ donation? Describe the criteria for organ donation.
2. What organs in this case, may be considered as suitable?
3. Describe, in detail, the legal requirements of consent by the next of kin for organ donation. If the patient was to be

referred to the Coroner or the Procurator Fiscal, would this prevent organ donation?

4. If the family agrees to donation, what would be the role of the transplant coordinator?

Answers

1. This patient would be an ideal candidate for organ donation.
   (a) He is otherwise well and the intracerebral lesion originates within the central nervous system.
   (b) His diabetes would not exclude donation of any organs as long as at retrieval he was found not to have extensive vessel disease.
   (c) As long as the second set of brainstem death tests confirm death and the relatives do not have any objection, organs may be removed for the purposes of transplantation.

   General criteria
   (a) There must be a confirmed diagnosis of brainstem death, as described by the code of practice (Working Party, 1993).
   (b) There must be no previous history of malignancy. The exceptions are primary brain tumours, since they do not metastasize outside the central nervous system.
   (c) The patient must be hepatitis B and human immunodeficiency virus (HIV) negative and may not fall within high-risk groups. This includes intravenous drug abusers, known homosexuals and prostitutes, where virology status may be difficult to determine.
   (d) The patient must be maintained on a ventilator.
   (e) There must be no unidentified or untreated sepsis.
   (f) For solid organ donation the patient must be <75 years old. For tissue donation a patient may be considered from any age group.
   (g) The following may *not* exclude a patient from donating organs:
      (i) A history of hypertension.
      (ii) Diabetes mellitus.
      (iii) Current identified sepsis.
      (iv) Previous hepatitis B.

(v) Positive hepatitis C virology.
(vi) Poor renal function; anuria; acute tubular necrosis.
(vii) High inotropic requirement.
(viii) Previous episodes of cardiac arrest.
(ix) Smoking or drinking.

2.

Suitable organs

(a) *Heart*

The electrocardiogram (ECG) should be within normal ranges with no evidence of infarction.

Chest X-ray should be normal.

If there is no prior history of cardiac disease.

Hearts will be considered from patients up to 60 years old.

(b) *Lungs*

If the chest X-ray is normal and lungs are radiologically clear, both lungs could be transplanted. If one lung is infected the other may be considered for a single-lung transplant.

If the arterial blood gases remain within normal ranges.

If there is no evidence of pulmonary infection at the time of the retrieval operation.

Lungs will be considered from patients up to 60 years old.

(c) *Kidneys*

There are very few contraindications to kidney donation. Slight elevation of the urea and creatinine in a normally healthy man would not exclude donation.

His diabetes would be noted on the kidney form but would not necessarily exclude transplantation.

Kidneys will be considered from patients up to 75 years old.

(d) *Liver*

If liver function is within normal ranges. (This *must* take into account changes that may be attributed to trauma or cardiac arrest.)

There should be no history of chronic alcoholism.

The normal markers for assessing liver function are the AST and ALT results. In patients where cardiac arrest or trauma has occurred it is expected that these may be deranged and therefore abnormal results would *not* exclude donation.

Low albumin may suggest a chronic liver failure but is assessed in conjunction with treatment of the patient from admission, as large infusions of crystalloid would also lower the albumin.

The transplant team assessment of acute liver failure may involve a request for a prothrombin time evaluation as elevation may indicate acute failure.

The acceptability of a liver for transplantation involves not only assessment of liver function but also requires an overview of the patient's treatment since admission as well as past history.

Livers will be considered from patients up to 75 years old. Parameters will vary as patient in fulminant hepatic failure require urgent transplantation, thus all organs will be considered.

(e) *Corneas*

If there is no history of previous intraocular surgery.

Corneas are considered from patients of any age. Diseases of unknown aetiology are a contraindication. Malignancy is not a contraindication, apart from lymphoblastic leukaemia, due to its unknown aetiology.

(f) *Heart valves*

If the heart were to prove unsuitable at the retrieval operation the aortic and pulmonary heart valves may be removed.

The only contraindication would be any evidence of valve disease.

Malignancy is not a contraindication to donation.

Valves can be donated from patients aged 6 months to 65 years.

(g) *Bone*

As long as the patient has no history of rheumatoid arthritis or sepsis, bone may be removed. In this case tendons may also be taken.

Bone is suitable for donation from patients of any age. Local policy will dictate the age limits for tendon donation, but in general may be considered up to 45 years.

(h) *Skin*

Due to the lack of long-term storage facilities in the UK, skin is taken when required for local plastic surgery or burns units.

Skin may be taken from patients up to 70 years old.

(i) *Pancreas*
This man would not be a suitable pancreas donor as there is a history of diabetes mellitus.

Pancreas may be transplanted from donors ranging from 12 to 55 years.

3. The Human Tissues Act 1961 enables a person lawfully in possession of the body to give permission for organs to be removed if, having made such reasonable inquiry as may be practicable, there is no reason to believe either that the deceased had expressed an objection to his or her body being so dealt with (or had not withdrawn it) after death or that the surviving relatives of the deceased object to the body being so dealt with (Department of Health and Social Security, 1975).

The guidelines *Cadaveric Organs for Transplantation* (Department of Health and Social Security document) state that if a patient carries a signed donor card or has recorded his or her wishes, there is no *legal* requirement to establish lack of objection on the part of the relatives, although it is good practice to take into account their views.

The guidelines state that relatives need only make known their lack of objection to donation and are not required by law to sign any documentation. If they wish to sign, the form should not be worded as consent but as lack of objection.

Material for research may only be removed at the retrieval operation if the relatives have given specific permission.

(a) *The practice of elective ventilation.* In early 1994 the Kings Fund Report *A Question of Give and Take* reported elective ventilation to be an unlawful practice as it was not directly performed for the benefit of the patient (New *et al.*, 1994).

(i) *Definition of elective ventilation.* Where a patient is admitted to hospital in a condition that will lead to certain death, a decision is made, with the full agreement of the next of kin, to ventilate the patient once respiration has ceased, for the sole intention of organ donation.

The Department of Health, following legal advice, has recognized that such treatment is initiated prior to death and cannot be described as being in the best interests of the patient. It is therefore illegal.

(ii) If the patient is to be referred for Coroner's post-mortem, it is necessary to obtain the authority of the Coroner for the removal of any part of the body.

Under the Home Secretary's direction, Coroners must act within the legal framework of this country but are not to make moral or ethical decisions in this matter. The Coroners should assist rather than hinder the procedure for organ removal. A Coroner should refuse consent only where there might be later criminal proceedings in which the specific organ might be required as evidence, or if the organ itself might be the cause or partial cause of death or where its removal might impede further enquiries (Brazier, 1992).

4. The transplant coordinator acts as an intermediary between the transplant teams and the patient considered for organ donation, his or her family and the staff in the donating hospital.

The practices of coordinators vary across the country but in general they will:

(a) Confirm suitability of an individual being considered for organ donation. This is often useful to establish before discussion with the family.
(b) If the family wishes, discuss the process of the donation and document their wishes regarding which organs and tissues are to be donated.
(c) Organize the virology testing of the organ donor (as well as obtain consent for testing from the family). The tests performed will be:
    (i) HIV surface antibody.
    (ii) Hepatitis C surface antigen.
    (iii) Hepatitis B surface antigen.
    (iv) Cytomegalovirus status.
(d) Advise on the principles of donor management.
(e) Request specific testing to allow the placement of organs.
    (i) Full biochemistry screen.
    (ii) Full haematology screen.
    (iii) Liver function testing.
    (iv) Chest X-ray
    (iv) ECG.

(f) In discussion with UK Transplant Authority and local transplant teams, place each organ prior to its removal, in accordance with national guidelines and the Human Organ Transplant Act 1989.
(g) Arrange operating theatre space and anaesthetic staff.
(h) Coordinate the arrival of each transplant team.
(i) Write to the family to thank them and to give them some details of the recipients whilst maintaining patient confidentiality.
(j) Write to all staff involved in the donation procedure.

In addition to the role at the time of donation, the transplant coordinator's role encompasses education to all members of the medical and nursing profession involved in the area of donation.

References

Brazier M. (1992) *Medicine, Patients and the Law.* Penguin, Hardmondsworth. pp. 405–406

Department of Health and Social Security. (1975) HSC 15 (156)

New B, Solomon M, Dingwall R and McHale J. (1994) A question of give and take. Improving the supply of organs for transplantation. *Kings Fund Institute Research Report* **18:** 64–65

Working Party on behalf of the Health Departments of Great Britain and Northern Ireland. (1983) *Cadaveric Organs for Transplantation. A Code of Practice Including the Diagnosis of Brain Death.* Department of Health and Social Security, London. pp. 33–39

Claire Hornick

Case 11 Hypertension and the surgical patient

A 46-year-old man was referred to casualty as an emergency by his general practitioner with acute abdominal pain in the right iliac fossa. He also gave a vague history of precordial discomfort and mild breathlessness on exertion for some months. He had stopped smoking 2 years previously, having smoked up to 40 cigarettes daily, and admitted to drinking 30 units of alcohol each week. The past history of note was a 4 year history of hypertension for which he was receiving nifedipine 20 mg twice daily. On examination the abdomen was soft with mild guarding in the right iliac fossa. His pulse was 96 beats/min and the blood pressure was 167/100 mmHg (phase V). A tentative diagnosis of acute appendicitis was made and he was admitted for observation.

Questions

1. When you examine the patient fully on the ward, describe the important physical signs you would search for.
2. What additional investigations would you perform?
3. How would you manage this hypertensive patient?
4. Discuss the treatment of hypertension.

Answers

1. Hypertension is defined as an abnormal elevation of the blood pressure, usually as a result of increased peripheral resistance. However, there is no universally accepted definition of the condition, and although the World Health Organization defines hypertension as systolic blood pressure greater than 160 mmHg and/or diastolic blood pressure of 95 mmHg or more, other factors such as age are not considered. The diagnosis is made by sphygmomanometry and in up to 10% of cases is secondary to renal or endocrine disorders.

Your examination should pay particular attention to the abnormal physical signs which influence prognosis. These include assessment of the central venous pressure, the presence of left ventricular hypertrophy (position of apex beat and fourth heart sound on auscultation), signs of left ventricular failure (basal crepitations) and hypertensive retinopathy. Renal masses must be sought and body habitus should enable Cushing's syndrome and acromegaly to be eliminated as causes.

2. The central venous pressure was normal. The heart was moderately enlarged clinically with the apex beat in the sixth intercostal space in the anterior axillary line. On auscultation there was a soft fourth heart sound and there were a few fine bilateral basal crepitations. The liver was not palpable and there was no peripheral oedema. Urinalysis was normal. The electrocardiogram (ECG) confirmed sinus rhythm with electrical left ventricular hypertrophy. The heart was enlarged on chest X-ray, with minor upper lobe blood diversion indicating pulmonary venous hypertension. The full blood count was normal and the urea 9.1 mmol/l and creatinine 173 μmol/l.

   Hypertension is usually asymptomatic and indeed, symptoms are often due to the development of complications. Only 30% of hypertensive patients have evidence of cardiovascular disease when the hypertension is first detected and 50% of patients with moderate hypertension (diastolic blood pressure >110–120 mmHg) have ECG criteria for left ventricular hypertrophy (LVH). The presence of LVH is associated with an impaired prognosis, with a 12-fold increase in risk of stroke and a threefold increase in intermittent claudication compared to normal people of the same age.

3. Sympathetic activity with arteriolar constriction elevates blood pressure (cf. phaeochromocytoma) and adequate analgesia is important. As the central venous pressure is normal, and the patient has basal crepitations, the increase in urea and creatinine is *not* due to dehydration but reflects pre-existing renal impairment as a complication of the hypertension. The presence of heart failure in association with LVH indicates the need for careful attention to fluid balance. Nifedipine is negatively inotropic and as such is not ideal for this patient. The most appropriate drug would be an angiotensin-converting enzyme (ACE) inhibitor, but

the patient's treatment should not be changed until the surgical management is clearer. The hypertension will respond to a combination of bedrest and abstinence from alcohol but it may be necessary to increase the nifedipine dose and add a low dose of a loop diuretic.

4. The treatment of hypertension should always be done cautiously unless there is an overwhelming need for immediate reduction in blood pressure, such as in pre-eclampsia. General measures should always be commenced first if possible, including weight reduction and restriction of salt and alcohol intake, but drug therapy is usually required. Treatment must be tailored to the individual patient and should be commenced using a single agent. There are no firm rules regarding which drug to use initially and the trial evidence points to the reduction in blood pressure as most important. Simplicity should be the keyword, and adequate dosage of one drug should be employed before a second is added. In patients awaiting elective surgery (such as herniorrhaphy) hypertension should be treated and the blood pressure returned to normal for a couple of months before the operation. The drugs used will to some extent be dictated by whether the patient has concomitant disease such as asthma (precluding a beta-blocker) or intermittent claudication (warranting care if a beta-blocker is considered). ACE inhibitors are now increasingly being used early in the management of hypertension but particular care must be taken in patients with peripheral vascular disease due to the association with renal artery stenosis. Any patient whose renal function deteriorates after commencing an ACE inhibitor must be considered to have renal artery stenosis and appropriate investigations (such as a diethylenetriaminepentaacetic acid (DTPA) renogram) should then be performed.

The range of drugs available to treat hypertension is constantly increasing, with the angiotensin II receptor antagonists being the latest addition to the therapeutic armamentarium. Regular monographs and editorials are published in the major medical journals regarding the treatment of hypertension and use of these drugs, and these should be consulted in preference to cardiology textbooks. The best option however is to consult a cardiological colleague for advice!

Further reading

Braunwald E. (ed.) (1991) *Heart Disease: A Textbook of Cardiovascular Medicine*, 4th edn. WB Saunders, Philadelphia

Leatham, Bull, Baimbridge and Leech. (eds) *Lecture Notes on Cardiology*, 4th edn. Blackwell, Oxford

David P. Dutka

Case 12 Arterial embolism and embolectomy

A 75-year-old man was admitted with a 4-h history of sudden onset of severe persistent pain in his left foot. He said that 1–2 h after the onset of the pain he lost the feeling in his toes and his foot became very cold. He had had no previous similar problems and led an active life with no leg symptoms. On examination his radial pulse was irregular and an electrocardiogram confirmed that he was in atrial fibrillation. There was some decrease in temperature distal to his left knee; the left foot was cold and pale, the veins were collapsed. There was hypoaesthesia distal to the ankle but no motor impairment. There were no peripheral pulses palpable distal to the left femoral pulse. All peripheral pulses were present in his right leg.

Questions

1. What is the differential diagnosis?
2. What are the aetiology and pathogenesis of the arterial lesion?
3. What is the place of heparin in the treatment of peripheral arterial emboli?
4. Describe with full operative detail the operation of femoral embolectomy.

Answers

1. The main condition that may be confused with peripheral embolism is acute arterial thrombosis of a diseased and stenotic artery. Occasionally acute thrombosis may be the complication of a peripheral aneurysm. The distinction between embolism and thrombosis is important to determine the treatment, because more extensive surgery is required for thrombosis and thrombectomy will often fail.

   Certain points from the history and clinical examination suggest thrombosis rather than embolism. A patient with a peripheral embolism has a sudden onset of symptoms with an identifiable source of an embolus, most likely of cardiac origin. Usually the proximal and contralateral pulses are normal. Typically, patients with thrombosis have a history of intermittent claudication and absent pulses, or reduced pressures in the contralateral limb. The degree of ischaemia is usually less profound in thrombosis, with preservation of skin sensation due to an established collateral circulation. The absence of heart disease further supports the diagnosis of thrombosis.

In doubtful cases an arteriogram should be performed. In patients with acute thrombosis diffuse atherosclerotic changes may be present, with well-developed collaterals and an irregular cut-off at the site of vascular occlusion. In contrast, angiographic findings of minimal atherosclerosis with few collaterals and a sharp cut-off, occasionally with a reversed meniscus, suggest an embolic aetiology. The location of the occlusion may also help to differentiate between embolism and thrombosis. An occlusion centred in the adductor canal usually indicates thrombosis while embolic occlusions are localized in arterial bifurcations. However, as a result of the proximal and distal propagation of the clot these findings may be obscured.

Other conditions that may be confused with peripheral embolism are aortic dissection, phlegmasia cerulea dolens, neurological disorders and low-flow syndrome due to circulatory failure.

2. The heart is the main source of emboli, resulting from atrial fibrillation, mitral stenosis or myocardial infarction.

   Atrial fibrillation may be the consequence of coronary artery disease. Thrombus forms because of stasis in the large fibrillating atrium. Emboli may follow the induced, or spontaneous conversion to, sinus rhythm. With mitral stenosis thrombi may be formed in the enlarged atrium as a result of restriction of flow; the problem may be accentuated by the commonly coexistent atrial fibrillation. Thrombi can also be formed on the damaged endocardium of the left ventricle after myocardial infarction. When embolism occurs its frequency is greatest in the first 2–3 weeks after the infarction, and in some patients it is the initial manifestation of a silent myocardial infarction.

   Other unusual causes of emboli are shown in Table 12.1.

3. Following the acute arterial obstruction by a peripheral embolus, proximal and distal thrombus propagation may occur, producing worsening of the ischaemia. Also, in cases of prolonged ischaemia, associated venous thrombosis may

Table 12.1 Sources of arterial emboli

The heart
Atrial fibrillation
Mitral and aortic valves
- Prosthetic
- Rheumatic
- Endocarditis

Myocardial infarction
Left ventricular aneurysm
Congestive cardiac failure
Cardiomyopathy
Atrial myxoma

The arteries
Atheromatous embolism
- Aorta
- Stenosis in iliac or femoral arteries

Thrombus from aneurysms
- Popliteal aneurysm
- Aortic aneurysm
- Others, rarely

The veins
Paradoxic embolus (a thrombus arising in the venous circulation passes through a congenital atrial or ventricular septal defect and lodges in a peripheral artery)
Tumour
Foreign body
Fragments of arterial catheters
Bullets entering major arteries

Unknown source
In 5–10% of cases the source of an embolus cannot be determined clinically or at autopsy

occur, probably from a combination of venous stasis and ischaemic damage to the endothelium.

As soon as the diagnosis of embolism is made, a bolus of 5000–10 000 units of heparin should be given, followed by a continuous intravenous infusion to reduce the secondary propagation of thrombus. This is carried on postoperatively in order to reduce the incidence of recurrent emboli and any arterial thrombosis due to endothelial damage from the embolectomy catheter. Although the adoption of this policy will increase in the incidence of wound haematomas, these rarely require reoperation and this risk is small in relation to the benefit of an increased patency and a significant reduction of recurrent emboli.

The incidence of recurrent emboli ranges from 6% to 45% in reported series. Oral therapy with warfarin begins on day 3 or 4 after surgery and continues for as long as the patient is at risk. Patients with intractable atrial fibrillation should stay on anticoagulation indefinitely while those with myocardial infarction should be treated for several weeks, by which time the endocardium will have healed and the likelihood of recurrent embolism is small.

4. As the patient is usually in a poor medical condition, often with a myocardial infarction, femoral embolectomy is performed under local anaesthesia using lignocaine 0.5–1%. Epidural anaesthesia is contraindicated if the patient is heparinized. Close monitoring during the procedure by an anaesthetist is recommended.

A vertical incision in the groin is used, exploring the common, superficial and profunda femoral arteries. Elastic slings are passed around these arteries. Following the embolectomy, atraumatic clamps are necessary to control the restored blood flow.

Either a transverse or a vertical arteriotomy is performed in the common femoral artery. A vertical arteriotomy is preferable in a diseased femoral artery as it gives better access to branches for catheter manipulation. It can also be used if a profundoplasty or a bypass procedure becomes necessary. A small incision is first made with a number 11 scalpel blade and the arteriotomy is enlarged longitudinally for 1.5–2 cm just proximal to the orifice of the profunda, using fine-angled scissors.

Generally a number 4 embolectomy catheter is used for distal exploration. The balloon must be tested before use. The embolectomy catheter is advanced in turn into the superficial femoral and profunda arteries. Embolectomy in the profunda should be restricted to 25 cm. The balloon is inflated and pulled back by the same surgeon, so that resistance can be felt and excess pressure not applied, since this can produce intimal damage. The procedure is repeated until no residual embolic material is extracted. After restoring good back-flow the distal arteries are flashed with heparin–saline solution. Although the amount of back-bleeding is not necessarily a good indicator as to how much of the embolic material has been removed, a total absence is a serious finding. It may indicate distal secondary thrombosis and an on-table angiography is indicated, to determine the extent of obstruction, and whether reconstruction is indicated. A small flush of blood flow proximally is released to dislodge any clot that may have been formed behind the clamps. If normal forward flow is not present, a number 6 embolectomy catheter could be passed proximally to remove any arterial or iliac embolus. The arteriotomy is closed with a continuous non-absorbable vascular suture.

In all cases histological examination should be requested for the embolic material for verification of the aetiology. After the arteriotomies are closed the distal clamps are removed first, followed by proximal, and haemostasis is checked. Good flow is indicated by the appearance of distal pulses, the filling of the peripheral veins and the return of the colour of the skin to almost normal. If there is any doubt, an intraoperative arteriography should be performed.

Further reading

Lumley JSP. (1986) *A Colour Atlas of Vascular Surgery*. Mosby-Wolfe, London

John Lumley
George Geroulakos

Case 13 Infantile groin swellings

A female infant aged 9 months was seen in the outpatient department with a swelling in the right groin. This has been noted intermittently for 4 weeks and is not increasing in size. On examination the swelling is non-tender and reducible.

Questions

1. Discuss the differential diagnosis.
2. What are the complications of the commonest of these diagnoses?
3. Describe your management, including operative details.
4. Which rare syndrome should be considered and what is its management?

Answers

1. The differential diagnosis includes an inguinal hernia, femoral hernia or hydrocele of the canal of Nuck. With this history the most likely diagnosis is an indirect inguinal hernia, especially if the swelling extends in the direction of the labium. Direct inguinal hernias are rare. Femoral hernias are also uncommon and, when present, appear below and lateral to the pubic tubercle. A hydrocele transilluminates and is typically difficult to reduce.

   Inguinal hernias in females may contain the ovary and fallopian tube, which are usually present as sliding elements.
2. Incarceration, with or without strangulation of the contents, is the main complication of an inguinal hernia in a female. In the absence of extreme tenderness and skin changes, manual reduction should be attempted as in males. If reduction is unsuccessful, urgent operative intervention is mandatory. The blood supply to the ovary can be compromised by incarceration or strangulation and ovarian atrophy can take place.
3. As the risk of incarceration is maximal in under-1-year-olds, a herniotomy under general anaesthetic should be performed within a few weeks. Through a 2-cm incision in the

groin crease, the anterior wall of the inguinal canal is displayed ad opened for a short distance along its length. On opening the canal the hernial sac with the adherent round ligament becomes visible. The sac should always be opened and the contents inspected because of the increased incidence of a sliding hernia. If the sac is empty, the neck is transfixed and the sac and the round ligament divided distally. If gonadal structures – usually ovary and fallopian tube – are seen they are carefully inspected. If the gonad is dysmorphic, a biopsy should be taken. If a sliding hernia is present, the sac is trimmed back and the edges oversewn just distal to the enclosed structures. The wound is closed in layers and the skin with an absorbable subcuticular suture.

There is a general consensus that contralateral exploration in girls is justified due to the high incidence of bilateral hernial sacs (50%) and the very low incidence of damage to reproductive organs.

4. In girls, the presence of bilateral hernias, a dysmorphic gonad or the absence of the uterus should alert one to the possibility of the testicular-feminizing syndrome. In this condition, infants have a 46,XY karyotype, a female phenotype and normal external female genitalia. The gonads are testes and are usually intra-abdominal but may descend into the inguinal canal. There is a blind-ending vagina with an absent uterus. It is estimated that 1 in every 200 females having a herniotomy has this condition and it results from male hormone insensitivity. Affected patients should always be reared as females. The testes should be removed during childhood, since there is a 4% incidence of testicular tumours by the age of 25 years and about 33% by 50 years. Oestrogen replacement therapy will be necessary at the age of puberty.

Further reading

Johnstone JMS. (1994) Hernia in the neonate. In: *Surgery of the Newborn*, 1st edn, Freeman NV, Burge DM, Griffiths M and Nalone PSJ (eds) Churchill Livingstone, Edinburgh, pp. 321–330

Imran Mushtaq
David P. Drake

Case 14 Gangrene

A 60-year-old man was brought to casualty complaining of a painful bullous lesion on his buttock and having felt shivery and nauseated for the past 12 h. He was a non-insulin-dependent diabetic but had no other past medical history of note. On examination, he was anxious and in pain. His temperature was 39°C. An oedematous area of purplish discoloration was noted over the right buttock. At the periphery of the area, crepitus was felt which extended over the buttock and the upper third of the right thigh; 1 ml of clear fluid was aspirated from the centre of the discoloured skin and sent for urgent microscopy and culture. The results of the microscopy were as follows: no pus cells and numerous Gram-positive rods.

Questions

1. Discuss the most likely diagnosis.
2. What is the significance of no pus cells seen in the microscopy of the aspirate?
3. How would you manage this patient?
4. What is the prognosis?
5. Discuss the epidemiology of this infection.

Answers

1. The rapid onset, pain, anxiety, bullous lesion, crepitus and Gram-positive rods in the aspirate suggest a diagnosis of gas gangrene. The most commonly isolated species of *Clostridium* in gas gangrene is *C. perfringens*, which accounts for approximately 80% of cases. However, other species of *Clostridium* may be implicated and these include *C. septicum*, *C. novyi* and *C. histolyticum*. It is not unusual to find more than one species of *Clostridium* involved in gas gangrene. In addition, gas gangrene frequently involves other species of bacteria, including *Escherichia coli*, *Proteus* spp., staphylococci and streptococci.

   Other conditions may produce similar clinical features to those described in this case, including gas formation.

Organisms which may be implicated particularly in mixed infections, include enterococci, *Klebsiella*, *Enterobacter*, *Escherichia coli*, staphylococci, streptococci, *Pseudomonas* and *Bacteroides* spp. However, none of these produce the massive muscle necrosis which is the characteristic feature of gas gangrene. The muscle changes are best seen at operation. Initially the muscle is pale but later becomes brown or purplish in colour. When incised, it is non-contractile and only bleeds slightly or not at all. Some gas may be present at this stage. Later, as the myonecrosis becomes more extensive, the muscle becomes friable and deep purple or black in colour.

2. The lack of inflammatory cells in the aspirate is typical of gas gangrene. *Clostridium* produces numerous exotoxins. These include lecithinases such as *C. perfringens* alpha-toxin and *C. novyi* gamma toxin. The effect of these enzymes is to damage or destroy cell membranes. This results in cell lysis. Therefore, in gas gangrene neutrophils are lysed, which is why they are scanty or absent in aspirates.

   Also, the lecithinases increase the permeability of capillaries. This results in oedema around the affected area and this compromises the blood supply, reducing the availability of white cells to the area.

   Lecithin is an important component of many tissues and the effects of lecithinases are widespread. The clear appearance of the aspirate, rather than being blood-stained, is probably as a result of lysis of red blood cells. This may in turn lead to intravascular haemolysis and haemoglobinuria. The destruction of platelets as a result of lecithinase activity may result in thrombocytopenia.

3. (a) *Surgical debridement.* The most important aspect of the management of gas gangrene is urgent surgical debridement of all affected tissues and thus the removal of most of the infecting organisms. This may involve amputation of a limb, removal of a limb or abdominal muscles or, in cases of uterine involvement, hysterectomy. The mortality rate in patients with gas gangrene without surgical intervention is virtually 100% and delays in surgical treatment are associated with a fatal outcome. Closure of the wound should be delayed until it is clear that infection is no longer present. Reoperation on a daily basis may be necessary to remove all necrotic tissue.

Debrided tissue should be sent for culture. This will help confirm the diagnosis. Also, it will enable the isolation and identification of other species of bacteria which may be contributing to the infection. Antimicrobial therapy may need to be altered depending on the culture results.

(b) *Antimicrobial therapy.* Antimicrobial agents are a useful adjunct to surgical treatment. Combination therapy should be administered intravenously to cover not only *Clostridium* but other organisms which may be involved in the infection, such as coliforms, enterococci, streptococci and other anaerobic bacteria such as *Bacteroides* spp. Penicillin is generally considered to be the antibiotic of choice against *Clostridium.* It should be combined with metronidazole which, as well as being active against *Clostridium*, is useful to treat other anaerobic bacteria. To cover aerobic bacteria which may be involved, an aminoglycoside such as gentamicin is usually added to extend the spectrum of activity. In patients who are allergic to penicillin, possible alternatives include erythromycin, vancomycin and chloramphenicol.

Before the widespread availability of antimicrobial agents, gas gangrene antitoxin was administered. The clinical response was extremely variable and there was a high incidence of allergic reactions. Gas gangrene antitoxin is no longer used or commercially available.

(c) *Hyperbaric oxygen.* Hyperbaric oxygen therapy may be given if available, although there are few clinical data available supporting its use. Hyperbaric oxygen increases the oxygen tension at the site of the infection, preventing anaerobic infection and toxin production. However, it is of less importance than surgical debridement and antimicrobial therapy in the treatment of gas gangrene. Its use does not justify the risk of delaying surgery or of transporting a critically ill patient to administer this treatment.

4. The overall mortality in patients with gas gangrene is approximately 25%. However, the prognosis varies depending on several factors, including the patient's age, the anatomical site involved and the stage at which the patient presents. Elderly patients have a worse prognosis than young patients. Patients who develop gas gangrene of a

limb following trauma have a survival rate of 90%. The clinical features of the case described here suggest spontaneous gas gangrene, which is associated with an increased mortality compared with gas gangrene following trauma. Gas production is a comparatively late finding and this suggests a worse prognosis. Involvement of the abdominal wall is also associated with a high mortality of between 50 and 60%. This is usually because its development is unexpected and it is difficult to recognize initially. Other poor prognostic features include shock at presentation, leukopenia, evidence of intravascular haemolysis and renal failure. Underlying conditions such as cancer or uncontrolled diabetes are also associated with a poor outcome. Features associated with a poor prognosis in gas gangrene are summarized in Table 14.1.

Table 14.1 Features associated with a poor prognosis in gas gangrene

Elderly patient
Underlying conditions
  Malignancy
  Diabetes mellitus
Spontaneous or postoperative
Abdominal or thoracic involvement
Long incubation period (>30 h)
Shock
Leukopenia
Haemolysis
Renal failure

5. Gas gangrene has been historically linked with war injuries. *C. perfringens* frequently contaminates war wounds, though only a small percentage develop gas gangrene.

   In peacetime, gas gangrene may follow trauma (50%), surgery (30%) or may occur spontaneously (20%; non-traumatic). Most cases of gas gangrene following trauma occur after major trauma such as road traffic accidents, penetrating injuries or severe burns. However, minor injuries such as simple cuts, insect bites or intramuscular injections may result in gas gangrene. Postoperative gas gangrene may occur and most commonly follows abdominal surgery. Uterine gas gangrene may follow septic abortion or, very rarely, a normal delivery.

Spontaneous gas gangrene occurs in patients with underlying conditions. Up to two-thirds of these cases are found to have diabetes mellitus.

Patients with malignant tumours, especially haematological malignancies and tumours of the colon, may present with gas gangrene. This clinical presentation is most commonly associated with *C. septicum.* It is unclear why this should be, since this species appears to be an unusual inhabitant of the human gastrointestinal tract.

Clostridium is widely distributed in nature and can be cultured from virtually all environmental sites, including operating theatres. However, most infections are associated with the patient's own *Clostridium*, although hospital outbreaks have occasionally been described.

Further reading

Case Records of the Massachusetts General Hospital (Case 46 – 1990) *New England Journal of Medicine* **323:** 1406–1412

Gorbach SL. (1992) Gas gangrene and other clostridial skin and soft tissue infections. In: *Infectious Diseases*, Gorbach SL, Barlett JG and Blacklow NR (eds). WB Saunders, Philadelphia, pp. 764–770

Pauline Jumaa
Soad Tabaqchali

Case 15 Renal transplantation

A 47-year-old woman with chronic renal failure as a result of glomerulonephritis has been on maintenance haemodialysis for $3\frac{1}{2}$ years. At 10.30 a.m. a cadaveric kidney is offered for her. The kidney was removed at 11.30 p.m. the previous evening from a 55-year-old man with a history of mild hypertension who died as a result of intracellular haemorrhage. The liver was also removed from the donor for transplantation.

Questions

1. What are the principles of kidney preservation and for how long may a kidney be stored?
2. The operation takes place in the standard fashion, the kidney being transplanted into the right iliac fossa. What surgical complications may present in the first 10–14 days postoperatively?
3. What surgical complications may present in the first year postoperatively?
4. What immunosuppressive drugs could be used?
5. What are the main complications of these drugs?
6. What are the main factors influencing long-term (say 5-year) graft survival in renal transplantation?

Answers

1. Preservation is normally accomplished by perfusion of the kidney at the time of donor nephrectomy, followed by storage in ice at approximately 4°C. Most perfusion solutions in clinical use are based on an intracellular electrolyte composition, with a relatively high potassium concentration (80–120 μmol/l) and a relatively low sodium concentration (9–80 μmol/l). To this are added a variety of other agents, including electrolytes, an osmotic agent to render the solution hyperosmolar and a number of intracellular metabolic precursors. A variety of solutions is available commercially. Of particular interest is the University of Wisconsin solution,

which has been shown to confer advantages for non-renal organ preservation – i.e. the liver and pancreas – and also provides excellent renal preservation.

Continuous machine perfusion is rarely used unless very long-term storage is anticipated. It is cumbersome, time-consuming and expensive. If the kidney is removed in ideal circumstances the limit to storage time is about 60–120 h.

Cadaveric kidneys are never removed in absolutely ideal conditions. Brain death causes a variety of endocrine changes to occur and many donors are haemodynamically unstable. There is likely to be a period of time when the kidneys are ischaemic before they are cooled, although *in situ* cooling may reduce this time to virtually zero.

Total storage time is a combination of this initial warm ischaemic time (WIT) and the cold storage time, and in general the longer the WIT, the shorter should the total storage time be. If WIT is less than 5–10 min, storage for 48 h or more may be acceptable. Initial WIT of greater than 30–45 min increases the risk that the kidney will never function post-transplant. There is increasing evidence that immediate graft function and medium-term graft survival are improved if total storage time is kept below 24 h.

2. (a) *Renal artery complications*
   - (i) *Thrombosis.* The incidence of renal artery thrombosis should be no higher than 1%.
   - (ii) *Haemorrhage.* Major arterial haemorrhage rarely occurs in the absence of significant infection at the site of the anastomosis.

   (b) *Renal vein thrombosis.* This occurs in up to 5% of renal transplants and, whilst it may follow technical complications – the vein may be twisted, stretched or compressed – there have been suggestions that it is more common following the introduction of cyclosporin. Presentation is typical – sudden loss of renal function associated with severe local pain around the site of the transplant. The kidney becomes swollen and there is perinephric bleeding which may be severe if the cortex of the kidney ruptures. Transplant nephrectomy is almost invariably required.

   (c) *Urinary tract complications*
   - (i) *Urinary leak.* Urine may extravasate from the ureter, the site of the ureterovesical anastomosis or the

bladder. Technical failures account for a proportion of urinary leaks but of more significance are the complications that follow ureteric ischaemia. The transplant ureter is dependent for its blood supply on vessels running alongside it from the renal artery. Ischaemia may result if the ureteric adventitia is stripped at the time of donor nephrectomy or transplantation. Severe ischaemia may cause necrosis of the ureter, leading to urinary extravasation.

(ii) *Lymphocele.* Lymph may leak from divided lymphatics in the kidney or from perivascular lymphatics divided during mobilization of the iliac vessels. Lymphoceles rarely occur in the first 2 weeks post-transplantation.

(iii) *Ureteric obstruction.* This may result from technical failure, oedema or haematoma at the uretero-vesicle anastomosis, or external compression from haematoma or lymphatic collections. The use of an indwelling JJ ureteric stent minimizes these complications.

3. (a) *Renal artery stenosis.* The incidence depends upon the number of renal arteries, the presence or absence of an aortic patch and the surgical techniques used. The incidence of clinically significant stenosis is reported to vary from 1.5 to 7%. The cause may be technical, result from trauma to the wall of the renal artery during perfusion, or may be associated with rejection.

   (b) *Ureteric obstruction.* Lesser degrees of ureteric ischaemia (not causing necrosis – see above) may result in progressive fibrosis of the lower end of the ureter leading to stricture formation.

   (c) *Lymphocele.* The peak time for the presentation of a lymphocele is 1–6 months post transplantation. Lymph collects and forms a cystic swelling typically between the lower pole of the kidney and the bladder. This may obstruct the ureter and may also compress the iliac vein causing ipsilateral leg oedema. Treatment is by aspiration/drainage followed by marsupialization into the peritoneal cavity if indicated.

4. (a) *Cyclosporin.* Introduced in 1983 cyclosporin (Sandimmun) has become the principal immunosupressive agent in virtually all transplant centres. Concerns about variable absorption and the effects of bile and food have

led to the recent introduction of a new formulation of cyclosporin, Sandimmun Neoral. The drug acts primarily on T helper lymphocytes, blocking the production of various cytokines of which Interleukin-2 is the most significant. The generation of cytotoxic T-cells is thus prevented. The initial dose of cyclosporin is usually 8–10 mg/kg/day, with maintenance doses (reached at 6–12 months) of 3–5 mg/kg/day.

(b) *Steroids.* While some transplant units use cyclosporin alone the majority combine it with 1 or 2 other agents with different mechanisms of action. Prednisolone is usually given in a dose of 20–30 mg daily initially, reducing to maintenance doses of 7.5–10 mg daily. Withdrawal of steroids 3–12 months post transplant has been shown to be possible for the majority of patients although some patients may experience a rejection episode following steroid withdrawal.

(c) *Azathioprine.* Following initial enthusiasm for the use of cyclosporin mono-therapy, or of cyclosporin + prednisolone, 'triple therapy' containing all three agents has become one of the most widely used regimens. The dose used ranges from 1–2 mg/kg/day.

(d) *FK 506.* This is the most recent immunosuppressive agent to come into clinical practice. Although most of the early experience has been in liver transplantation a number of centres have treated kidney recipients with the drug. Its mode of action is very similar to that of cyclosporin.

(e) Several other drugs have been used experimentally and in clinical trials. Most promising of these appears to be Mycophenolate mofetil, which blocks purine synthesis, and early clinical trials suggest that this is an effective drug in reducing the incidence of acute rejection.

(f) Antibodies; both polyclonal and monoclonal anti-lymphocyte preparations are used by many centres for prophylaxis or for the treatment of vascular (or steroid-resistant) rejection. Anti Lymphocyte Globulin (ALG) and Anti Thymocyte Globulin (ATG) are polyclonal whilst the most commonly used monoclonal antibody is OKT3.

5. (a) *General side effects*

(i) *Infection.* Ideal immunosupression would produce immunological tolerance. Current drug therapy is not specific to the transplanted kidney and is required ad infinitum. Non-specific depression of the immune system renders the recipient more susceptible to infection. In general the more immuno-suppression used (and in particular the greater the use of the various antibody preparations) the greater the risk of infection. Bacterial infections (wound, urinary tract, blood) are the most common infective processes in the immediate posttransplant period. Viral, fungal and protozoal infections have a higher incidence 1–12 months posttransplantation.

(ii) *Cancer.* Several large international tumour registries have shown clearly that there is a highly significant increased risk of some, but not all, cancers. Tumours with the greatest increased incidence are those of skin and the lymphatic system, where the increased risk may be several hundred times that of the general population. It has become increasingly apparent that those tumours known or suspected to be associated with viral infections are amongst the most common in transplant recipients.

(b) *Specific side-effects*

(i) *Cyclosporin.* The major side-effect of cyclosporin that is relevant in clinical practice is nephrotoxicity. This may be acute – haemodynamically mediated and reversible on dose reduction – or chronic – associated with marked interstitial fibrosis and probably not reversible. Early fears that long-term maintenance therapy with cyclosporin was likely to lead to progressive and inevitable renal impairment have not been borne out by clinical experience in renal transplantation. Other side-effects of cyclosporin include hypertension, tremor, hirsutism, gingival hyperplasia and hyperuricaemia.

(ii) *Steroids.* The list of side-effects of steroids is extensive and well-documented. In renal transplantation the doses used are relatively low and thus the side-effects are relatively minor. The most significant include hypertension, hyperglycaemia, Cushingoid features, osteoporosis and growth retardation in children.

(iii) *Azathioprine.* Bone marrow suppression, liver dysfunction and non-malignant skin tumours may occur.

6. Many factors influence renal transplant outcome. These include donor factors (age, cause of death, comorbidity), kidney factors (multiple renal arteries, quality and duration of perfusion), recipient factors (age. primary renal disease, blood transfusions) and immunological factors (pretransplant human leukocyte antigen (HLA) sensitization, HLA matching and immunosuppressive regime). Some of these factors influence immediate and short-term graft survival, whereas others are only apparent in longer-term follow-up studies.

   Death with a functioning transplant (primarily from cardiovascular disease) becomes increasingly important as older patients are more widely considered to be suitable transplant recipients.

   (a) *Patient survival.* The operative mortality associated with renal transplantation has fallen to less than 1%. Patient survival at 1 year is approximately 90–95% and at 5 years about 80%.

   (b) *Graft survival*

   (i) *Living donors.* The best results are achieved with HLA-identical living donor transplants. Both 1- and 5-year graft survival are over 90%. With non-identical living donors 1-year graft survival is still over 90% but 5-year graft survival falls to about 75–80%.

   (ii) *Cadaver donors.* The influence of HLA matching on graft survival in cadaveric renal transplantation has become clear from large international registries. These have shown that, whilst 1-year survival (approximately 80–85%) is only marginally influenced, 5-year results are clearly correlated with HLA matching. HLA-identical grafts have a 5-year survival of 70% or more, whereas totally mismatched grafts result in a 20–25% inferior outcome. Intermediate matching produces intermediate results, with the strongest influence being matching at the Dr locus.

Further reading

Morris PJ. (1994) *Kidney Transplantation: Principles and Practice*, 4th edn. WB Saunders, Philadelphia

Christopher John Rudge

Case 16 Gastric cancer

A 44-year-old heavy goods vehicle driver presented to his general practitioner with a 2–3-month history of epigastric pain which was relieved by eating and also by ranitidine therapy. He had lost at least 10 kg in weight over the preceding 12 months. There was no relevant previous medical history; in particular, there was no history of previous dyspepsia or other gastrointestinal disease. He smoked 20 cigarettes a day and had a 10–20-unit alcohol consumption per week. There was no family history of gastrointestinal cancer.

He was referred to hospital for further investigation and had an upper gastrointestinal endoscopy which showed generalized erythematous gastritis and a small localized area of irregular mucosa close to the incisura. Biopsies of this area were taken and showed evidence of signet-ring adenocarcinoma. He proceeded to operation, when the only abnormality found was of slight thickening of the gastric wall in the region of the incisura. A total gastrectomy with excision of the greater and lesser omentum was performed. Reconstruction was by an oesophagojejunostomy Roux-en-Y.

He made a good postoperative recovery and was discharged 11 days following surgery. Histology showed adenocarcinoma of the stomach of intestinal type confined to the mucosa and submucosa of the lesser curve. Resection margins were clear of tumour and there was no evidence of lymph node metastasis.

Questions

1. What are the indications for upper gastrointestinal endoscopy in patients with dyspepsia?
2. What is the incidence of gastric cancer?
3. What are the treatment options for a patient with gastric cancer?
4. What pathological types of gastric cancer occur and how are these tumours staged?
5. What is the prognosis for patients who have had a 'curative' resection of a gastric cancer?
6. How may the population be screened for gastric cancer and are such screening programmes effective?

Answers

1. In many young patients or those with an established diagnosis, upper gastrointestinal endoscopy is unnecessary before commencing therapy for dyspepsia. However, new dyspeptic symptoms in a patient aged 40 years or older is an indication for endoscopic assessment. The majority of these patients will have a diagnosis established and up to 2% will be found to have a gastric carcinoma. For other patients associated symptoms such as vomiting, weight loss and dysphagia or a family history of gastric carcinoma are also indications for endoscopy. Severe symptoms or those that fail to respond to conventional therapy should also prompt investigation.

   Endoscopy may also be used to establish the presence of *Helicobacter* infection, particularly if eradication therapy is contemplated. However, there are alternative, less invasive techniques for the diagnosis of *Helicobacter* infection, including a breath test.
2. Approximately 15 patients per 100 000 population in England and Wales are diagnosed as having gastric cancer each year. Over the years there has been a slight decline in the incidence of this condition associated with an increased proportion of proximal (cardia, fundus and upper-body) tumours. There is wide variation in the incidence of this disease worldwide, with a particularly high incidence found in south-east Asia.
3. A tissue diagnosis obtained by endoscopic biopsy would normally be followed by liver scanning (ultrasound or computed tomography (CT)) to identify any metastatic disease. In the absence of metastases patients considered suitable for operation would normally be offered resectional surgery. Operative options include oesophagogastrectomy (for cardia tumours invading the lower oesophagus), total gastrectomy (with oesophagojejunal anastomosis), subtotal gastrectomy (removal of approximately seven-eighths of the stomach, leaving a small proximal gastric remnant for anastomosis to the jejunum), distal gastrectomy (suitable for patients with localized antral or pyloric tumours) and proximal gastrectomy (with oesophagoantral anastomosis) – an operation which has become less popular in recent years. All of these resectional operations are associated with clearance of local lymph nodes in the greater and lesser omentum.

The extent of the lymph node excision will depend on the stage of the tumour and its position. There has been considerable debate about the value of radical lymph node excision, and although the results of further trials are awaited, it appears that extensive lymph node dissection (so-called R_2 or R_3 operations) is associated with increased operative morbidity and mortality for relatively little, if any, survival benefit. The spleen, distal pancreas and transverse colon may also require excision in some cases to achieve local tumour clearance. The jejunum may be brought up for anastomosis either as a simple loop or more commonly as a Roux-en-Y; some surgeons construct a jejunal reservoir to act as a new stomach. For patients with gastric outlet obstruction and locally advanced or metastatic disease a gastrojejunostomy may be performed to relieve obstruction.

Endoscopy may also be used to treat gastric cancers. There are some reports of laser or diathermy excision of early gastric cancers through the gastroscope. For obstructing lesions, laser therapy or intubation is possible as palliative treatment for those with metastatic disease or unfit for major operation. The recent introduction of expanding metal stents has facilitated endoscopic intubation of lesions causing obstruction at the oesophagogastric junction.

Recent chemotherapy studies using a combination of epirubicin, cisplatin and continuous 5-fluorouracil infusions have shown encouraging responses in patients with inoperable disease. This combination of chemotherapy is currently being used in a perioperative chemotherapy trial (Magic study). Radiotherapy is occasionally used for the treatment of local or regional disease.

4. Macroscopically these tumours may be ulcerative (65%), diffusely infiltrating (25%) or fungating (10%). Microscopically they are divided into two types – the intestinal type, which shows a glandular pattern, and the diffuse or signet-ring (mucin-containing) tumours. Mixed tumours showing both types of differentiation occur. Other malignant gastric tumours occur, including lymphomas, leiomyosarcomas and, less commonly, secondary deposits, particularly from malignant melanomas.

The TNM classification of gastric cancer as modified in 1987 is shown in Table 16.1.

Table 16.1 TNM staging of gastric cancer

	TNM stage		
Stage			
I	T1N0M0	T1N1M0	T2N0M0
II	T1N2M0	T2N1M0	T3N0M0
IIIa	T2N2M0	T3N1M0	T4N0M0
IIIb	T3N2M0	T4N1M0	

T1 = Confined to mucosa/submucosa.
T2 = Invading muscularis propria to subserosa.
T3 = Through serosa.
T4 = Through serosa with involvement of contiguous structures.
N0 = No nodal involvement.
N1 = Affected nodes <3 cm from tumour.
N2 = Affected nodes >3 cm from tumour.
M0 = No distant metastases.

Early gastric cancer is usually defined as tumour confined to the mucosa and submucosa irrespective of lymph node or metastatic status. The 5-year survival for these patients is greater than 90% following resection.

5. The prognosis is stage-dependent. Stage I tumours are associated with a 90% 5-year survival following successful resection, compared with 70% for stage II tumours and 30% for stage III tumours.

   Multivariant analysis of prognostic factors has shown that distant metastasis, the depth of tumour invasion through the gastric wall and the presence of lymph node metastasis are independent variables for a poor prognosis.

   The operative mortality for resection of gastric cancers has been high in the past, reaching 20 or 30% in some series. More recent studies from the UK and abroad have shown operative mortalities of less than 5%. Part of the explanation for this is improvements in perioperative management in patients who are often elderly with other medical problems.

   The increasing use of upper gastrointestinal endoscopy and particularly the availability of open-access endoscopy services has led to a shift towards earlier stage of tumour at diagnosis, associated with increased resection rates and improved prognosis.
6. Endoscopic surveillance for the development of gastric dysplasia and cancer is effective. A national screening programme has been established in Japan for over 10 years and

a carcinoma is found in approximately 1 in every 1000 endoscopies. Almost half of these tumours are early gastric cancer at the time of diagnosis and 98% of these screen-detected tumours come to operation. Because of the lower incidence of gastric cancer in the UK, endoscopic screening programmes are extremely expensive, but early investigation of dyspeptic symptoms and surveillance of those at high risk of developing gastric cancer, such as those with dysplasia or a strong family history, are recommended.

Further reading

Inokuchi K. (1981) Evaluation of extensive lymph node dissection for carcinoma of the stomach. *World Journal of Surgery* **5:** 241–248

Robertson C, Chung S, Woods S, Griffin S, Raines S, Lau J and Li A. (1994) A prospective randomised trial comparing R_1 sub-total gastrectomy with R_3 total gastrectomy for antral cancer. *Annals of Surgery* **220:** 176–182

Sue-Ling H, Johnston D, Martin I *et al.* (1993) Gastric cancer: a curable disease in Britain. *British Medical Journal* **307:** 591–596

Jeremy N. Thompson

Case 17 Testicular cancer

A 30-year-old man presented to his general practitioner with a 3-week history of a left-sided scrotal swelling. It was painless, and the patient was certain that it had not been present any longer than 3 weeks. The general practitioner examined the swelling and found a hard irregular swelling which was non-tender and located in the lower part of the left testicle. The general practitioner referred the patient for a surgical opinion.

Questions

1. What is the differential diagnosis?
2. What are the commonest pathological types of testicular tumours and how are they staged clinically?
3. What are the tests which should be performed on this patient to stage his disease accurately?
4. What should be the surgical approach to this patient?
5. Describe the treatment of testicular tumours and relate this to their clinical stage.

Answers

1. Scrotal swellings can be divided into two groups on the basis of their presentation – acute or chronic.
   (a) Acute scrotal swellings
      (i) Acute epididymo-orchitis.
      (ii) Testicular torsion.
      (iii) Haematocele with or without testicular rupture.

      In the young patient it is impossible to differentiate between infection and torsion, and it is not worth taking the risk. It is possible that colour Doppler ultrasound may help in doing this, but once again, the time it may take to do this test and the risk that it may be wrong do not justify a conservative approach. A young patient under the age of 25 who presents with such an acute lesion without a history of trauma will require immediate scrotal exploration.

The patient with a haematocele will, of course, have a history of trauma. Scrotal examination will be important in this group also, particularly in the presence of two situations: first, if the swelling is large and likely to cause pressure on the testicle which may lead to future atrophy, and second, if the tunica albuginea is ruptured with extrusion of testicular tissue. This can usually be diagnosed on scrotal ultrasound. If exploration of the traumatized testicle is undertaken, and rupture is found after the blood has been aspirated and necrotic testicular tissue removed, the tunica can be closed with a 3-0 absorbable suture.

(b) Chronic scrotal swellings
   (i) Cystic
      Hydrocele.
      Spermatocele.
      Epididymal cyst.
      Cyst of the spermatic cord.
   (ii) Solid lesions
      Infective (tuberculosis, gumma).
      Tumours of the testicle.

When confronted with a chronic swelling of the testis, the key part of the physical examination is transillumination, which will without fail differentiate between solid and cystic lesions. If the lump is found to be solid, a scrotal ultrasound may be helpful, but tumour markers (alpha-fetoprotein, beta human chorionic gonodotrophin; beta-hCG) should be tested.

2. The commonest types of testicular tumours are seminoma and non-seminomatous germ-cell tumour (the latter was called teratoma in the past). There are a number of other different types of testicular neoplasms, such as Sertoli cell and Leydig cell tumours. In patients over 70, the commonest type of testicular tumour is a primary lymphoma of the testis. The most frequently used method of clinical staging of testicular tumours is the Royal Marsden staging:

Stage I: Tumour confined to testes.
Stage IIa: Para-aortic lymph node involvement less than 2 cm.
Stage IIb: Para-aortic lymph node involvement 2–5 cm.

Stage IIc: Para-aortic lymph node involvement greater than 5 cm.
Stage III: Supradiaphragmatic nodal involvement.
Stage IV: Visceral involvement.

3. The tests which should be performed are as follows:
   (a) Serum alpha-fetoprotein and beta-hCG. Unfortunately, there is no specific tumour marker for seminoma of the testis, but one or both of the above are elevated in 95% of cases of non-seminomatous germ-cell tumour of the testis.
   (b) Computed tomography (CT) scan of chest, abdomen and pelvis. The lymphatic drainage of the testes is directly to the para-aortic lymph nodes and then to the supradiaphragmatic nodes. The CT scan will thus accurately define enlarged nodes, giving details of their relationship to the inferior vena cava and aorta. In addition, it will be clearly seen if nodes are present above the renal arteries close to the crura of the diaphragm. If the nodes are compressing either urethra leading to hydronephrosis, this will also be seen without difficulty.

   The CT scan will also help in searching for visceral metastases either in the liver or the lung. A chest X-ray and serum liver function tests should also be done.
4. Preoperatively, the patient should be warned that an orchiectomy will be performed. If a testicular tumour is suspected, the operation should be performed through an inguinal incision. The incision is made from the skin markings of the deep inguinal ring to the pubic tubercle. The incision is extended through superficial and deep fascia to the external oblique muscle. This is then opened and the inguinal canal is thus entered. The spermatic cord is divided at the deep inguinal ring, with the proximal stump being suture-ligated with 2-0 chromic catgut. If there is considerable doubt in the mind of the surgeon, the spermatic cord can be cross-clamped at the level of the deep ring and the testicle delivered into the wound. This manoeuvre should only rarely be performed, and it is an absolute requirement that the venous drainage be blocked before the testicle be handled in order to prevent spread of tumour cells. After delivery into the wound the testicle can be examined more closely, and if necessary it can be bivalved. This latter manoeuvre should only be performed after great consideration,

as it is a consequence of this that the testicle may atrophy. It is clear that the surgeon should go into this operation with as much knowledge about the testicular lesion as possible. A frozen section on the table is rarely of use, as testicular tumours are usually most reliably diagnosed histologically by permanent paraffin sections, with an element of doubt existing on the assessment of the frozen sections.

The histological classification of testicular tumours is as follows:

Stage I Primary tumours
(a) Germ cell
(b) Specialized gonadal stromal
  (i) Leydig cell
  (ii) Sertoli cell
(c) Gonadoblastoma
(d) Miscellaneous
  (i) Mesenchymal
  (ii) Adenocarcinoma of rete testis
  (iii) Carcinoid
  (iv) Adrenal rest tumours
Stage II Paratesticular tumours
Stage III Secondary neoplasms

The British classification of germ cell tumours, described by Collins and Pugh in 1964, which differs somewhat from the American classification, is as follows:

1. Seminoa
   (a) Typical
   (b) Spermatocytic
2. Malignant teratoma
   (a) Undifferentiated (MTU)
3. Teratoma
   (a) Differentiated (TD)
   (b) Malignant teratoma intermediate (MTI)
4. Malignant teratoma
   (a) Trophoblastic (MTT)
5. Yolk sac tumour

The correct appellation of teratoma is non-seminomatous germ-cell tumour. Poor prognostic histological features are venous invasion or invasion of the cord. Carcinoma-*in-situ* describes a pattern of atypical germ cells seen in seminiferous tubules associated with invasive germ-cell tumours. It is associated with 85% of ipsilateral and 5% of contralateral testicles with seminoma and some types of non-seminomatous germ-cell tumours.

5. The recommended management stage by stage of testicular seminoma is as follows:
   (a) *Stage I:* This is the commonest stage of seminoma at clinical presentation of the disease. The optimal way of managing this is by giving low-dose radiotherapy (30 Gy) to the abdominal nodes. This will ensure a 100% 5-year survival rate for this stage. Alternative methods have been used, such as observation only and low-dose chemotherapy. At present these are under evaluation and cannot be considered superior to 30 Gy radiotherapy.
   (b) *Stage II:* Stage IIa and IIb are traditionally treated by full-dose (60 Gy) radiotherapy to the abdominal nodes. It has been shown that stage IIc is best treated by the use of chemotherapy. The reason for this is that the incidence of local recurrences of disease and the incidence of residual masses is much lower if chemotherapy is used. It is felt by some that chemotherapy should also be used in stage IIb.

      The chemotherapeutic schedule used in the treatment of nodal disease is referred to by the acronym BEP, consisting of bleomycin, etoposide and cisplatin. Six courses are given and then the patient is reassessed by checking the CT scan.
   (c) *Stage III:* The recommended treatment is chemotherapy with BEP.
   (d) *Stage IV* likewise: the optimal therapy is using chemotherapeutic agents as described above.

   The management stage by stage of non-seminomatous germ cell tumours is as follows:
   (a) *Stage I:* There are two schools of thought as to the best way of treating stage I non-seminoma. Observation and treatment when nodal metastases develop are effective in producing a 98–99% 5-year survival rate. If observation is chosen as the therapeutic strategy, subsequent nodal metastases will develop in 30% of patients. These are then given a full course of chemotherapy, generally with BEP.

The other option is to perform a primary retroperitoneal lymph node dissection. This involves complete clearance of the para-aortic lymph nodes from the crura of the diaphragm to the bifurcation of the common iliac arteries on both sides. It has recently been modified in an attempt to avoid retrograde ejaculation because of concomitant dissection of both sympathetic chains. The modification means that there is an extensive para-aortic nodal dissection on the side of the lesion with a less extensive dissection on the contralateral side, with preservation of the sympathetic ganglia and chains. This approach has resulted in preventing retrograde ejaculation in most cases.

Primary retroperitoneal lymph node dissection results in a similar 5-year survival rate as observation and chemotherapy if nodal metastases develop.

(b) *Stage II:* There are two schools of thought also in the management of stage II disease. It is felt appropriate by some to treat all stage II disease with chemotherapy using BEP. This usually results in excellent 5-year survival rates. If, after chemotherapy, there are residual masses noted on CT scan, a secondary retroperitoneal lymph node dissection is performed. In previous studies it has been found that when the residual masses are examined histologically, roughly one-third consist of fibrous or degenerative tissue, one-third consist of mature teratoma and one-third of residual tumour. In the latter two cases further courses of chemotherapy are required.

The other approach is to perform a primary retroperitoneal lymph node dissection in stage II disease followed by chemotherapy if the histology is positive. Once again, the 5-year survival rates are comparable to primary chemotherapy.

(c) *Stages III and IV:* These stages are treated by intensive chemotherapy with BEP.

It has been shown that the survival of non-seminomatous germ-cell tumour of the testis has been greatly improved by an aggressive combination of chemotherapy and surgery, as described above, in association with careful observation using CT scanning and tumour markers.

Further reading

Gleave ME and von Eschenbach AC. (1994) Testicular tumours. In: *Clinical Urology*, Krane RJ, Siroky MC and Fitzpatrick JM (eds). J.B. Lippincott, Philadelphia. pp. 1143–1175

John M. Fitzpatrick

Case 18 Cardiopulmonary resuscitation

A 62-year-old man was admitted to hospital with a painful swelling in his left groin. The man was fit and well (American Society of Anesthesiologist (ASA) grade I) and was diagnosed by the surgical registrar as having an obstructed inguinal hernia which required emergency surgery. Surgery was carried out at 03.00 h and a small direct hernia was found. There was no evidence of any obstructed viscus. The painful swelling was ascribed to some inflamed lymph glands. As recovery was closed overnight, the patient was returned directly to the ward at 05.00 h. At 06.00 h the cardiac arrest team was called to the patient who was found to be unconscious, apnoeic and pulseless.

Questions

1. What was the cause of postoperative collapse and cardiac arrest in this patient?
2. What is the incidence of complications occurring in the post-operative period?
3. What is the management of the patient who has had a post-operative cardiac arrest?

Answers

1. Recent multicentre studies of complications in the peri-operative and postoperative period have shown that 42% occur in the postoperative period and that the prognosis for these events was much worse than for any other time in the perioperative period. In one study 18 of the 40 perioperative cardiac arrests survived, whereas only 3 of the 19 post-operative cardiac arrest patients survived. Postanaesthetic respiratory depression was the commonest cause (46%), with inhalation of gastric contents (25%) the second commonest cause.

   A number of factors must be taken into consideration when considering the collapse of this patient. A relatively old man was undergoing emergency surgery in the early hours of the morning. A formal recovery area was not available and the patient's rapid return to the ward area, where less experienced staff and none of the sophisticated monitoring systems used routinely in postoperative monitoring (electrocardiogram, non-invasive automated blood pressure, pulse oximetry) were available. It is more than likely that this man suffered postoperative respiratory depression from an accumulation of opiate analgesics administered during and after the operative period. The resultant apnoea led to hypoxia and hypercarbia, resulting in a bradycardia and eventually asystole.

2. Figures of complications related to anaestheisa vary from study to study according to the historical date of the study and precisely what the authors were monitoring. In one study there were 449 cardiac arrests from 163 240 anaesthetics with an overall anaesthesia-related mortality of 0.9 per 10 000 anaesthetics. In the more recent studies carried out by Confidential Enquiry into Perioperative Deaths (CEPOD) there were 5081 deaths from 485 850 operations. CEPOD noted the following as increased risk factors (Buck *et al.*, 1987):

   (a) *Age.* Increased age was associated with higher risk. Some 75% of deaths were in patients aged over 70 and the authors commented that the margins for error were considerably narrowed in the older patient.

   (b) *Emergency versus elective surgery.* It was generally agreed that there was an increased risk of perioperative cardiac arrest in an emergency procedure over an elective one. One-fifth of the deaths in the CEPOD study were emergencies and 40% urgent procedures. The authors felt that more than 10% of these fatal operations were judged unnecessary.

   (c) *Inexperience.* CEPOD found that there was no consistency in the request to ask for an experienced surgical or anaesthetic opinion. In total, 21% of all operations, 29% of emergency operations and 45% of out-of-hours procedures were carried out without referral to a consultant surgical or consultant anaesthetic opinion.

   (d) *Monitoring.* The need for minimal standards of intraoperation monitoring is well-established (electrocardiogram, non-invasive blood pressure and pulse oximetry) but the postoperative recovery period is often ignored.

This is usually when medical staff are not immediately present, monitoring is minimal and patients are supervised as a group rather than on an individual basis. Some 50% of complications occur in the first postoperative hour, 75% within 5 h – thus extending the postoperative period well beyond most medical expectations.

(e) *ASA physical status.* The ASA is a widely used classification of the patient's physical status. It is therefore not surprising that there is a correlation between ASA grade and operative risk. CEPOD reported that 73.8% of emergency operations were ASA grade V. Of more concern was the report that half of the elective procedures were considered to be ASA grade V. We must conclude that some very-poor-risk patients were being subjected to elective surgery and dying subsequently.

3. Cardiopulmonary resuscitation must begin immediately on the discovery of an unconscious apnoeic and pulseless patient. The initial procedures are called basic life support.

   A – airway: Open the airway by head tilt, chin lift and/or jaw thrust. Clear the airway of secretions or foreign material by suction if necessary.
   B – breathing: If opening the airways has not allowed the patient to breathe, mouth-to-mouth (or mask) rescue breathing must commence. Place your mouth over the patient's mouth and seal the nose by squeezing it between two fingers. Alternatively place a resuscitation mask over the patient's mouth and nose, ensuring a tight fit and that the patient's airway remains open. Blow into the airway and watch the chest rise with each individual breath. Give two breaths. If the chest does not rise, then the airway must be repositioned and further attempts made to ventilate the patient.
   C – circulation: If there is no detectable carotid pulse, begin external chest compressions. These are carried out on the lower third of the sternum using the overlapping heels of both hands. In the adult 15 compressions are alternated with two ventilations if one rescuer is present; five compressions are alternated with one ventilation for two or more rescuers. The compression rate is approximately 80/min and the depth of compression is 4–5 cm in the normal adult.

In hospital the cardiac arrest team must be called immediately, on discovery of the patient who has no pulse and is not breathing. They should, on arrival, find basic life support being attempted. The team will then:

A – airway: secure the airway by intubation of the trachea.
B – breathing: ventilate the patient using a bag-valve mask and oxygen reservoir system providing 60–80% oxygen-enriched expired air.
C – circulation: establish venous access with a wide-bore venous cannula and establish a definitive cardiac diagnosis by monitoring the electrocardiogram.

These rhythms are closely associated with cardiac arrest and the management algorithm for each is shown in Figure 18.1.

(a) *Outcome.* Basic life support (mouth-to-mask ventilation with external chest compressions) was in progress when the cardiac arrest team arrived. When the patient was attached to the electrocardiogram the monitor showed asystole. Adrenaline (1 mg) was administered intravenously and basic life support continued. Because of the probability of postoperative respiratory depression being the cause of the collapse, naloxone, a narcotic opiate antagonist, was also administered intravenously. Shortly afterwards there was a return of spontaneous circulation. Following stabilization the patient was moved to intensive care where he was ventilated for a further 2 days. On the third day he was removed from the ventilator and on day 5 he was returned to the high-dependency area. He was discharged home 14 days after admission to hospital and remained off work for another 6 weeks.
(b) *Conclusion.* Patients must be thoroughly investigated and proper formal opinions sought before embarking on surgical procedures at unsocial hours, especially where full operating room and recovery area facilities are not available on a 24-h basis.

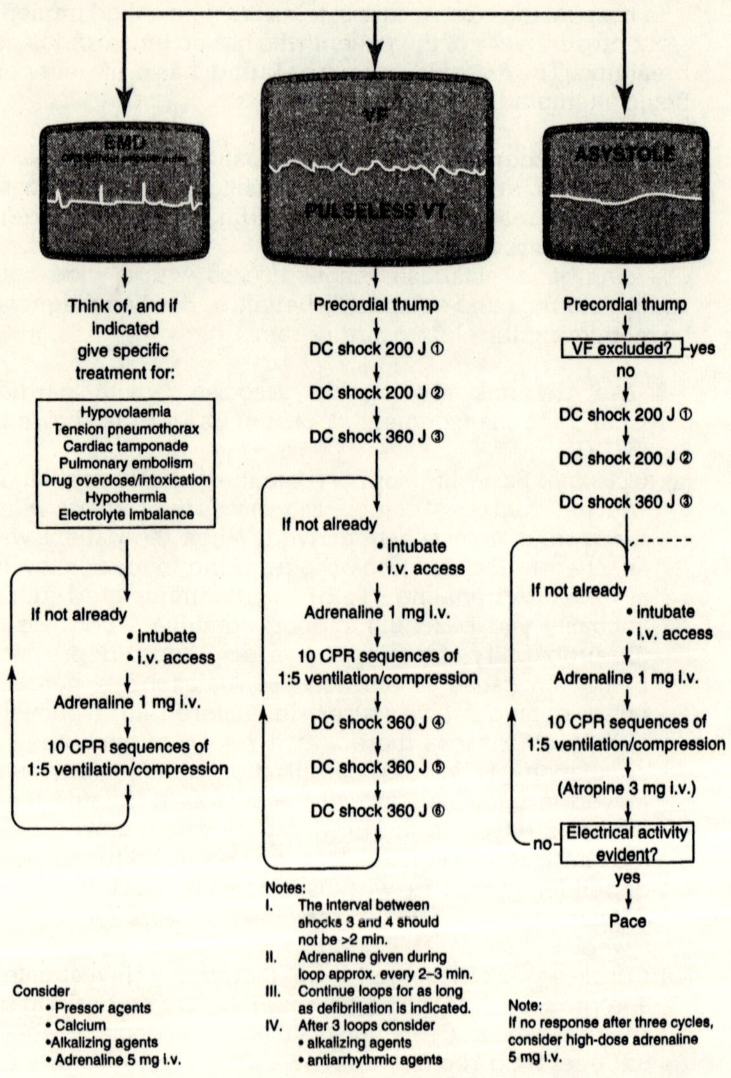

Fig. 18.1 Rhythms associated with cardiac arrest and management algorithm

References and further reading

Buck N, Devlin HB and Lunn JN. (1987) *The Report of a Confidential Enquiry into Perioperative Deaths (CEPOD).* Nuffield Provincial Hospitals Trust/ Kings Fund, London.

Colquoun MC, Handley AJ and Evans TR. (1995) *ABC of Resuscitation*, 3rd edn. British Medical Journal Publishing Group, London

D.A. Zideman

Case 19 Scoring on the intensive care unit

A 30-year-old man was admitted to hospital following a road traffic accident. He had sustained a closed head injury (Glasgow Coma Score (GCS) 7 on arrival in the accident and emergency department) and fractured ribs 5–10 on the right side causing a flail segment. A right underwater seal chest drain was inserted. He was intubated and ventilated and transferred for a computed tomography (CT) scan which revealed a right-sided extradural haematoma in association with a skull fracture. He was taken directly to the operating theatre where the haematoma was evacuated. An intracranial pressure monitor was inserted.

He was taken from theatre to the intensive care unit (ICU), where ventilation was continued with muscle relaxation and sedation. Chest X-ray revealed increasing shadowing underlying the flail segment, suggestive of significant lung contusion. By the following morning he was requiring an F_{IO_2} of 70% to maintain a Pa_{O_2} of 10.0 kPa. Other observations and investigations revealed:

Temperature	37.8 °C
Pulse	105 beats/min regular
Blood pressure	115/70 mmHg
Respirations	12 (ventilated) breaths/min
pH	7.36
Pa_{CO_2}	3.6 kPa
Haemoglobin	10.7 g/dl
White blood cells	14×10^9/l
Na	134 mmol/l
K	4.5 mmol/l
Cr	96 mmol/l

His intracranial pressure increased progressively, reaching 21 mmHg. Following a stat dose of mannitol intravenously in an attempt to lower the intracranial pressure a pulmonary artery (Swan–Ganz) catheter was inserted to guide fluid management in view of his severe head injury and lung contusion.

Despite continuing active management on the ICU, his condition continued to deteriorate. Three days later he remained ventilator-dependent on 100% oxygen. He was pyrexial 38.5°C, and was requiring inotropes to maintain his blood pressure. He had developed acute renal failure. He died from multiple organ failure 2 weeks later.

Questions

1. What are prognostic scoring systems? Which prognostic scoring systems could be used to predict outcome for this patient and how do they compare?
2. The neurosurgical unit manager informs you that there is a shortage of ICU-trained nurses for the next shift. Which scoring system would you use to determine the nursing dependence of this patient and how is the score calculated?
3. What simple clinical assessment might enable you to assess this patient's prognosis 6 days after admission to ICU?
4. It is suggested that the cost of intensive care in your unit is significantly higher and the outcome worse than that in other units. How could you use scoring to compare the efficacy and efficiency of the care provided by your unit with that provided by others?

Answers

1. Scoring systems can be used to stratify patients to their risk of requiring a particular intervention or of a particular outcome. Scoring systems should be objective and quantitative; they may address the extent of a specific disease or injury (cancer staging, burn indexes, abbreviated injury scale), the degree of dysfunction of a particular system (GCS, Ranson score), the amount of therapy required (the Therapeutic Intervention Scoring System; TISS) or the degree of physiological derangement (Acute Physiology and Chronic Health Evaluation (APACHE), the Mortality Prediction Model (MPM) and the Simplified Acute Physiology Score (SAPS)). Intensive-care patients are a heterogeneous group and outcome prediction often requires a generally applicable scoring system, rather than a disease-specific method, especially if comparisons are to be made across patient groups. However, for certain categories of patient, such as the patient described above, disease-specific scoring may be remarkably accurate.

Some workers have claimed that the GCS is a sensitive outcome predictor in acute head trauma, independent of other variables. Based on a prospective study of 1311 hospitalized head trauma patients in 1978, a GCS of 3 at time of admission predicted an 83% mortality; a GCS of 4–5 49% mortality; 6–7 (as in the patient described above) 24% mortality; and greater than 8, 0.3% mortality. Improved predictive accuracy may be achieved if the GCS is combined with other simple observations or diagnostic information such as pupillary reactivity. A recent study demonstrated that 75% of patients with unreactive pupils immediately following resuscitation died or were left in a persistent vegetative state compared with only 8.5% of those with reactive pupils.

The Injury Severity Score (ISS) and combined Trauma and Injury Severity Score (TRISS) were developed to predict survival in trauma patients across a wide range of severity of injury, but were not specifically tested in trauma cases requiring intensive care. TRISS has recently been evaluated in a group of 2414 critically ill trauma victims from six centres, and found to be inaccurate in this subset. Limitations of the TRISS methodology were identified and a revised model created, ASCOT (A Severity Characterization of Trauma), which was subsequently shown to be more reliable predictor of outcome. It is not clear, however, whether ASCOT has any advantages over APACHE III in predicting outcome in critically ill trauma patients.

The ISS has been used in important clinical trials in intensive care patients. Use of ISS to stratify patients according to risk of death enabled Watt and Ledingham to suggest a link between the use of etomidate as a sedative on the ICU and increased mortality after trauma. The drug was subsequently shown to be a potent inhibitor of adrenal steroidogenesis. This patient's ISS was 32 and trauma score 13, which gives a calculated probability of survival of 93%.

For patients in intensive care with multiple organ pathology, the disease-specific scoring systems are generally less accurate than those which have been designed for the heterogeneous ICU population. A number of scoring systems have now been described, and these generally address the degree of a patient's physiological derangement. The APACHE score is the most widely used and extensively validated of these systems. APACHE was first described in 1981 and refined in 1985 as APACHE II and again in 1989 as APACHE III. In this system points are allocated according to first, the degree to which a series of physiological variables (it is recommended that the worst value in the first 24-h period be recorded) differ from normal to derive an acute physiology score; second, age, and third, chronic health evaluation. APACHE III also considers the surgical status (elective versus emergency), the source of the patient prior to ICU admission and the admission diagnosis. The score is converted to a probability of hospital mortality using individual logistic regression equations for each of the diagnoses and patient origins. This patient's APACHE II score was 11, which converts to a probability of hospital mortality of 4%.

SAPS was developed in France from 13 of the 34 original physiological variables of APACHE. Data collection is therefore simplified but, unlike APACHE, the score does not incorporate information on diagnosis or the chronic health status of the patient and is perhaps for this reason less powerful than the updates of APACHE, APACHE II and III.

MPM produces a probability of mortality rather than a score, based on information recorded at the time of admission to intensive care. It has recently been updated as MPM II, which comprises two distinct models producing separate probabilities of hospital mortality on admission to the ICU and then at 24 h. Age and admission diagnosis and condition are required, along with a number of variables which are recorded as present or not present. As the information is obtained from admission data, the MPM probability estimate is independent of the effects of ICU treatment; however, the model is subject to the effects of lead time bias in that there is no allowance for the effects of treatments received before admission to ICU. As the model provides an assessment of severity of illness on admission to ICU, it may have advantages if the effects of early treatments on ICU are to be studied, and if stratification of patients before randomization into a clinical trial is necessary. MPM II is based on 19 000 patients from 139 ICUs spread across national borders, and has been shown to meet high standards for discrimination and calibration. It has, however, not been validated outside these centres.

2. The nursing dependence of an individual patient and the nursing requirements of a unit as a whole can be determined using TISS. TISS was first described in 1974 and

revised in the light of advances in ICU therapy in 1983. The system categorizes most therapeutic interventions in intensive care into one of four groups which are allocated scores of 1–4 on the basis of the significance of that intervention in relation to the severity of the patient's illness. For example, the need for controlled ventilation with muscle relaxation receives 4 TISS points, whereas supplementary oxygen therapy by mask receives only 1 TISS point. Ideally, TISS data are collected by a trained observer (usually an ICU nurse), preferably the same person each day, and at the same time of day. Points are allocated if the particular intervention occurred at any time during the previous 24 h. Where a patient has experienced more than one intervention affecting a particular body system, the intervention which attracts the highest TISS score should be selected. Total TISS points should decrease as the patient's condition improves. Total TISS points can be stratified into four groups:

Class IV	>40
Class III	20–39
Class II	10–19
Class I	0–10

Patients in class IV will require at least 1:1 nursing care. A trained ICU nurse would be expected to be able to look after one class III and one class II patient simultaneously. Four class II patients could be looked after by a single trained nurse with help from an auxiliary. Class I patients do not need intensive care. A patient with a total TISS score of >50 is likely to need more than one nurse's care for at least some of the time.

Although it is claimed that TISS can be used to determine severity of illness, it cannot be used for between-unit comparisons, since it is dependent on unit policies and the individual doctor's practice. For example, not every unit employs intracranial pressure monitoring in the routine management of acute head injury, and the use of pulmonary artery catheterization varies greatly between units. This patient's TISS in the first 24 h after admission was 47.

3. A number of studies have shown that the onset of multiple organ failure is a significant negative prognostic feature postsurgery or trauma. The greater the number of organ system failures and the longer their duration, the less likely the patient is to survive. The presence of three or more organ failures for greater than 5 days has been said to be

associated with 100% mortality. Multiple organ failure is common on the ICU, and patients can continue to survive in multiple organ failure with support for weeks, if not months, and few will recover. The presence of multiple organ failure a week after admission to ICU does, however, place the patient in a high-risk group and, taken with other features of the case, such as age and underlying diagnosis, may allow a physician to make a reasonable clinical estimate of prognosis.

4. Because patient populations differ considerably from one unit to another, crude comparisons of mortality rates and costs between intensive care units are an insensitive indicator of efficiency and quality of care. Generally applicable prognostic scoring systems such as APACHE II allow more meaningful comparisons between units, for example by comparing the predicted mortality with actual mortality to derive a standardized mortality ratio SMR. Such calculations may assist audit and lead to improvements in quality of care, as well as encouraging greater efficiency. TISS scoring can be used to calculate the cost of intensive care, although because TISS scoring cannot be used to compare severity of illness between units, such cost comparisons must be combined with an appropriate severity of illness score, as well as calculation of SMRs in order accurately to assess cost-effectiveness.

It is important to note that thus far we have concentrated on hospital mortality even though this is not necessarily the only outcome measure of interest. Length of ICU stay and subsequent hospitalization have important social and financial implications, whilst many would consider that the risk of significant disability, as well as subsequent quality of life, are equally important. They are, however, much more difficult to quantify, and are not assessed by currently available scoring systems.

TISS and severity of illness scoring can also be used to assess current utilization of a hospital's intensive care beds, as well as to predict future requirements. Risk prediction has also been used to identify patients who do not need intensive care, either because they are too sick or are not sick enough, thus releasing beds and reducing costs.

Further reading

Boyd CR, Tolson MA and Copes WS. (1987) Evaluating trauma care: the TRISS method. *Journal of Trauma* **27:** 370–378

Cullen DJ, Civetta JM, Briggs BA and Ferrera LC. (1974) Therapeutic intervention scoring system: a method for quantitative comparison of patient care. *Critical Care Medicine* **2:** 57–60

Keene AR and Cullen DJ. (1993) Therapeutic intervention scoring system: update 1993. *Critical Care Medicine* **11:** 1–3

Knaus WA, Draper EA, Wagner DP and Zimmerman JE. (1985) APACHE II: a severity of disease classification system. *Critical Care Medicine* **13:** 818–829

Knaus WA, Wagner DP, Draper EA *et al.* (1991) The APACHE II prognostic system: risk prediction of hospital mortality for critically ill hospitalised adults. *Chest* **100:** 1619–1636

Le Gall JR. (1995) Severity scoring in the critically ill patient. In: *Current Opinion in Critical Care*, vol. 1, Bone RC and Vincent J-L (eds). Current Science, Philadelphia, PA

Schuster DP and Kollef MH. (eds) (1994) *Predicting Intensive Care Unit Outcome. Critical Care Clinics.* WB Saunders, Philadelphia, PA

Michael O'Leary
Charles Hinds

Case 20 Paediatric burns

A 10-year-old child is admitted to the accident and emergency department with burns to the trunk and limbs following a fire. The respiratory rate is 60 breaths/min. The hospital has no burns units.

Questions

1. Discuss your initial management, with particular reference to the need to transfer the child.
2. What factors will determine the best time for transfer?
3. Describe the difficulties of interhospital transfer and how they might be overcome.

Answers

1. Obtain a history, and in particular the time of the burn and the materials involved (furniture, indoor or outdoor). Initial treatment must never be delayed whatever the child's initial appearance.

   Initial examination should determine the area of skin involved and the cardiovascular state of the child. Facial burns, perioral oedema, soot in the mouth and respiratory distress all point to inhalation injuries. Other injuries sustained by the mode of burn (collapsing burning building, car fire following collision) should be excluded.

   The child should be weighed. Blood should be taken for full blood count, cross-match, urea and electrolytes, carbon monoxide and cyanide levels. A chest X-ray should be performed.

   One large infusion should be started using full aseptic precautions. The use of a central vein improves security of the line, especially for transfer, and allows the cannula to be left *in situ* longer, as well as facilitating measurement of central venous pressure. Several fluid regimens exist, but the overriding consideration is to give adequate volumes rather than debate on the merits of differing types of fluid.

   Fluid regimens are based on the area of burn, and include the rules of nine, Lund and Browder charts and the Parkland regime. Divide the time from the burn into three periods of 4 h. In each period give x ml of plasma protein fraction:

$$x = \frac{\text{Area burned} \times \text{weight in kg}}{2}$$

Use blood instead of fresh frozen plasma if haematocrit falls below 0.3. Estimate the circulating blood volume (80 ml/kg for children) and give 1% of this for each 1% of burn, usually in the second 4-h period.

Third, give 2 ml/kg per h of water as 5% dextrose.

The efficacy of the regime should be assessed hourly by monitoring urine output (catheterize the bladder), haematocrit and cardiovascular parameters.

Inhalation injuries require expert assessment. Upper-airway injury is most common and can produce rapid total obstruction in children. Injury to the tracheobronchial tree occurs in one-third of inhalational injuries, resulting in bronchospasm and infection, whilst damage to the respiratory unit occurs in 5% of cases, resulting in reduced oxygen and carbon dioxide transport.

Early respiratory distress requires careful intubation. The presence of laryngeal oedema may necessitate the use of smaller than normal endotracheal tubes, and intubation should normally be performed nasally. Securing the tube is vital before transfer and can be taxing in the presence of facial burns. The gases must be humidified and physiotherapy commenced.

Analgesia is simpler in the intubated child because respiratory depression can be managed by intermittent positive-pressure ventilation. In the unintubated child, morphine can be given intravenously and titrated against effect, watching for a reduction in respiratory rate. Pulse oximetry and attempts to assess pain levels are of much less value.

The burns should be cleaned and covered. Constricting eschars should be divided. A major difficulty in transfer will be heat loss, and early aggressive heat conservation from admission is important. Convective body heaters are the best method of warming. All fluids should be warmed and all inspired gases humidified.

2. The benefits of transfer are to provide surgical and medical expertise for the burns. The child will also benefit from transfer if the referring hospital does not have paediatric

intensive care facilities. Transfer should under no circumstances be considered until the airway is secured and, if the child is intubated, ventilation should be commenced because of the difficulties of assessing respiration in transit.

3. Following adequate resuscitation, including correction of fluid deficit, acid–base disorders, respiratory distress and pain, the child should be set up for transfer. Minimum monitoring will include electrocardiogram (needle electrodes may be needed for attachment), pulse oximetry, blood pressure and temperature. End-tidal carbon dioxide measurement (capnography) is highly recommended.

   The child must be well-wrapped to conserve heat. The aircraft or ambulance should be prewarmed. All fluids should be warmed either by prewarming and use of an insulated box or by use of an exothermic gel cover to the fluid bag and giving set. A condenser humidifier is mandatory if the child is intubated.

   Blood should be available for the transfer. Pain should be controlled before departure, or if the child is intubated, full sedation must be instituted.

   The relatives must be informed of the transfer. One parent may be allowed to travel with the child if there is room, but the final decision is that of the transferring doctor. The risk of the child becoming frightened in transit must be considered and planned for.

   The receiving unit must be informed of the arrival time so that they are prepared. The child should be transferred to the burn unit before handover to minimize the risk of heat loss and infection.

Aubrey Bristow

Case 21 Brainstem death

A 25-year-old male was admitted to the intensive care unit with a severe head injury following a road traffic accident. He had a Glasgow Coma Score of 5 on admission to the accident and emergency department and a computed tomography (CT) scan of the brain revealed diffuse brain swelling with multiple small haemorrhages in both frontal poles. He had no other injuries and no relevant past medical history. An intracranial pressure (ICP) monitor was inserted and revealed an ICP of 19 cmH_2O. Medical management of his brain injury included moderate hyperventilation (to $Paco_2$ 3.8–4.2 kPa), maintenance of cerebral perfusion pressure and mannitol if the ICP exceeded 25 cmH_2O. The patient was sedated with propofol and paralysed with an infusion of short-acting muscle relaxant.

On the day following admission, the ICP remained high despite therapy with mannitol and increased doses of propofol. Infusion of dopamine was required to augment systemic blood pressure to maintain cerebral perfusion pressure. At 36 h after admission, when the ICP was 45 cmH_2O, both pupils suddenly dilated and became non-reactive. Repeat CT scan revealed gross cerebral swelling with obliteration of the ventricles. Sedation was discontinued and by the following morning the patient was still making no response. A tentative diagnosis of brainstem death was made and the patient prepared for formal testing of brainstem function. Relevant investigations at this stage showed:

Haematology:	Haemoglobin	10.9 g/dl
	white cell count	9.3×10^9/l
	platelets	180×10^9/l.
Biochemistry:	Na	163 mmol/l
	K	4.2 mmol/l
	urea	10.3 mmol/l
	creatinine	75 μmol/l
	and osmolality	329 mmol/kg.
Arterial blood gases:	Pao_2	16.3 kPa
	$Paco_2$	4.1 kPa
	pH	7.39.

Questions

1. May tests of brainstem function be carried out immediately? Describe the preconditions for the diagnosis of brainstem death.
2. How can residual effects of sedative and neuromuscular blocking drugs be excluded?
3. Describe the clinical tests which must be carried out to diagnose brainstem death. Are supplementary investigations necessary to confirm this diagnosis?
4. How often must the tests for brainstem function be carried out and by whom? What time interval is required between different sets of tests?
5. When does death occur?

Answers

1. This patient is hypernatraemic. The plasma sodium must be corrected prior to brainstem testing (see Principles of Donor Management, Case 10).

   Before testing for brainstem function takes place, the patient must be deeply comatose and the diagnosis certain and compatible with irreversible brain damage. Other causes of coma must be excluded and the following preconditions met:

   (a) Core temperature must be greater than 35°C. Active measures may be required to maintain normothermia as temperature regulation is markedly impaired after brainstem death (see Principles of Donor Management, Case 10).
   (b) Metabolic abnormalities must be excluded and, if present, corrected prior to testing. In particular hypo- and hypernatraemia, hypo- and hyperglycaemia, uraemia and hepatic encephalopathy should be considered.
   (c) Endocrine abnormalities must be excluded.
   (d) There should be no residual effects of alcohol or other sedative and neuromuscular blocking drugs.
2. Adequate neuromuscular function can be confirmed using a peripheral nerve stimulator. With the increased use of short-acting muscle relaxants administered by continuous infusion, there is rarely a need to reverse the effects of neuromuscular blocking agents.

Sedative drug effects in critically ill patients may however be more difficult to exclude. In this patient, propofol was used for sedation. This drug is rapidly metabolized and its duration of action is not prolonged in the critically ill. As over 12 h had elapsed between discontinuation of propofol infusion and testing for brainstem function, it can be safely assumed that there were no residual effects of this agent. However, if testing was required within a shorter period of time, plasma levels of propofol may usefully be measured, as they correlate well with the central effect of this drug.

Patients may also be sedated with benzodiazepines and opiates and both of these groups of drugs have active metabolites which are slowly excreted in critically ill patients. Plasma levels may be of little help in assessing residual effect, as plasma concentrations of benzodiazepines and opiates correlate poorly with central effect. Waiting adequate periods of time may establish the absence of drug effects, whereas the use of the benzodiazepine and opiate antagonists, flumazenil and nalaxone, provide pharmacological confirmation.

3. The examination to confirm the diagnosis of brainstem death should be carried out in accordance with the guidelines set out by the Conference of the Medical Royal Colleges and their Faculties in 1976. The clinical tests required to confirm the absence of brainstem function are:
   (a) Absent pupillary response to light.
   (b) Absent corneal reflex.
   (c) Absent motor response in the cranial nerve distribution in response to painful stimulation of the face, limbs and trunk.
   (d) Absent gag reflex.
   (e) Absent cough reflex.
   (f) Absent eye movement on caloric testing (at least 20 ml of ice-cold saline must be injected into each ear, having previously obtained a clear view of the tympanic membrane. The eyes must be observed for at least 30 s after injection of the saline).
   (g) No respiratory effort despite a $Paco_2$ >6.7 kPa in the presence of adequate oxygenation.

In the UK, clinical testing alone is acceptable to confirm the diagnosis of brainstem death. Absence of brainstem function is taken to be indicative of cessation of cortical function and formal testing is not required. In other countries, however, diagnosis of brainstem death requires the absence of cortical function to be verified by electroencephalogram confirmation of the absence of cortical electrical activity or an absent cerebral circulation during cerebral angiography.

4. The test for brainstem function must be carried out on two separate occasions to ensure that there is no observer error. Two doctors, normally the consultant in charge of the case and an independent consultant, must perform the tests for the diagnosis of brainstem death to be confirmed. In the absence of a consultant, any medical practitioner who has been fully registered with the General Medical Council for at least 5 years may carry out the tests for brainstem function. If the brainstem-dead patient is to become an organ donor, no member of the transplant team may be involved in testing.

   In the UK there is no proscribed time interval between the two sets of tests. The essential factor is that the tests must be carried out *independently* by two *different* medical practitioners. Although there is no legal requirements, it is often helpful to leave a period of time between the two sets of brainstem tests to allow discussion with the patient's relatives. This is often the time during which the subject of organ donation may be broached.
5. In the UK, brainstem death is confirmed at the time of the second test for brainstem function and this is the time of death. This is the case even if ventilation is continued for some time beyond the time of the diagnosis.

Further reading

Curry PD and Bion JF. (1994) The diagnosis and management of brain death. *Current Anaesthesia and Critical Care* **5**: 36–40

Health Departments of Great Britain and Northern Ireland. (1979) *The Removal of Cadaveric Organs for Transplantation: A Code of Practice*. HMSO, London

Health Departments of Great Britain and Northern Ireland. (1983) *Cadaveric Organs for Transplantation: A Code of Practice Including the Diagnosis of Brain Death*. HMSO, London

Honorary Secretary of the Conference of Medical Royal Colleges and their Faculties in the United Kingdom. (1976) Diagnosis of brain death. *Lancet* **ii**: 1069–1070

Honorary Secretary of the Conference of Medical Royal Colleges and their Faculties in the United Kingdom. (1979) Diagnosis of brain death. *Lancet* **i**: 261–262

Honorary Secretary of the Conference of Medical Royal Colleges and their Faculties in the United Kingdom. (1981) Diagnosis of brain death. *Lancet* **ii:** 365

Pallas C. (1983) *ABC of Brain Stem Death. Articles from the British Medical Journal.* British Medical Association, London

Martin Smith
Claire Hornick

Case 22 Acute lower limb thrombosis

A 69-year-old man was admitted to casualty with a 6-h history of sudden onset of severe pain distal to his right ankle. For the previous 8 months he had been experiencing intermittent claudication in his right thigh, calf and buttock at 200 m. He had also undergone coronary artery bypass graft 3 years previously. On examination his radial pulse was regular and there were no cardiac bruits. His right foot was cold and pale. There was a bruit over the right iliac artery with a decreased ipsilateral femoral pulse and no other pulses palpable below this level. On the left leg there was a bruit over the adductor canal; the popliteal pulse was decreased in amplitude and the posterior tibial pulse was absent.

Question

1. What is the differential diagnosis?
2. How will you perform an angiogram?
3. What is the treatment of acute arterial thrombosis?

Answers

1. The main condition that may be confused with acute arterial thrombosis is peripheral embolism. (For further details, see case 12.)
2. Percutaneous catheterization of the common femoral artery (first described by Seldinger in Sweden in 1953) is the catheter technique used by most radiologists. The patient is placed supine on the angiographic table and both femoral pulses are examined. The strongest is chosen for the arterial catheterization. If the pulses are equal the right is easier to catheterize by a right-handed operator standing on the patient's right side. Local anaesthetic is administered in the groin crease and in the soft tissues around the artery.

   A 2-mm incision is made with a number 11 scalpel blade at the skin entry point of the arterial cannula. The arterial cannula is advanced at an angle of 30–45° into the lumen of the femoral artery at a point which is approximately 2–5 cm below the inguinal ligament. A good pulsatile flow is obtained and the central stylet of the arterial cannula is removed. A curved-tip guidewire is then inserted into the artery through the cannula and advanced into the aorta. The function of the guidewire is to guide the catheter through the skin, the soft tissues and the arterial wall into the lumen of the artery, and then through the iliac system, the walls of which may be tortuous and stenotic, into the aorta. The cannula is next removed from the femoral artery and a size 4 F (1 F = 0.3mm) catheter is threaded over the guidewire and advanced into the aorta. The catheters contain insoluble metal salts to make them radiopaque. The type and amount of these additives also affect the stiffness of the catheter. Fluoroscopic monitoring allows exact positioning of the catheter.

When the catheter is correctly placed, the guidewire is removed. A test injection of a small amount of contrast is given under fluoroscopic monitoring, thus an adjustment can be made of the tip of the catheter to the desired location before the main injection. If the catheter needs to be advanced after the guidewire has been removed, the guide must be reinserted and the catheter advanced over it. The total volume of contrast medium used for an examination should not exceed 4–5 ml/kg; this is 350 ml for the average 70-kg patient.

3. When the diagnosis of acute thrombotic occlusion is made, intravenous heparin is instituted immediately and an arteriogram is performed. If on examination there is neurological deficit, this indicates that muscle necrosis is imminent and surgical exploration is the treatment of choice. A thrombectomy is rarely, if ever, useful in these acute arterial occlusions. A bypass graft is necessary and the type of bypass is tailored according to the angiographic findings. If on clinical examination there is no sensorimotor deficit the first-line therapy is percutaneous intra-arterial thrombolytic therapy. According to the guidelines of the consensus document of the National Institutes of Health (USA, 1980), contraindications for thrombolytic therapy include:
   (a) Absolute contraindications
      (i) Active internal bleeding.
      (ii) Recent (within 2 months) cerebrovascular accident or other active intracranial process.

(b) Relative major contraindications
  (i) Recent (<10 days) major surgery, obstetric delivery, organ biopsy, previous puncture of non-compressible vessels.
  (ii) Recent serious gastrointestinal bleeding.
  (iii) Recent serious trauma.
  (iv) Severe arterial hypertension (>200 mmHg systolic or >110 mmHg diastolic).

(c) Relative minor contraindications
  (i) Recent minor trauma, including cardiopulmonary resuscitation.
  (ii) High likelihood of a left heart thrombus, for example, mitral disease with atrial fibrillation.
  (iii) Bacterial endocarditis.
  (iv) Haemostatic defects, including those associated with severe hepatic or renal disease.
  (v) Pregnancy.
  (vi) Age over 75.
  (vii) Diabetic haemorrhagic retinopathy.

Thrombolysis should be avoided, using a knitted Dacron graft implanted in the retroperitoneal space, since occult bleeding may occur through the graft even many years following the initial surgery. The integrity of these grafts depends on thrombus incorporated in the interstices.

The most commonly used thrombolytic agents are streptokinase and tissue plasminogen activator (t-PA). There is controversy over whether systemic heparinization enhances the process of thrombolysis. Some studies have shown a beneficial effect for heparin, while others have shown no advantage. The mean infusion time for low-dose streptokinase or t-PA is between 20 and 30 h for most series (range 15–40 h). The dose of streptokinase is usually 5000 iu/h. Currently there is lack of consensus on the appropriate regime for t-PA. Our own practice is to give 0.5 mg/h. Several studies have shown that low doses of t-PA (0.5 mg/h) give low complication rates and equally high efficacy of lysis.

The management of the cause of the thrombosis is important because, unless the cause can be identified and treated, rethrombosis will occur. If an underlying stenosis of the superficial femoral artery is revealed then, after the completion of thrombolysis, an angioplasty should be performed. In some series approximately one-third of patients will require percutaneous transluminal angioplasty. If, however, after the completion of thrombolysis there is a persistent occlusion of the distal superficial femoral artery or the popliteal artery as a result of atherosclerosis or an aneurysm, a bypass graft is indicated.

Further reading

Lumley JSP. (1986) *A Colour Atlas of Vascular Surgery.* Mosby-Wolfe, London

Earnshaw JJ and Gregson RHS. (1994) *Practical Peripheral Arterial Thrombolysis.* Butterworth-Heinemann, Oxford

John Lumley
George Geroulakos

Case 23 Respiratory failure and oxygen therapy: ventilation and weaning

A 74-year-old man with a diagnosis of colonic carcinoma is admitted for laparotomy. He is noted to suffer from chronic obstructive airways disease (COAD) treated with salbutamol and ipratropium bromide inhalers and he is obese (weight 90 kg, height 150 cm). All laboratory results are within the normal range and the electrocardiogram is normal. The chest X-ray is constant with COAD and arterial blood gases on air are: pH 7.36; $Paco_2$ 5.8 kPa; Pao_2 10.1 kPa; HCO_3^- 25 mmol; base excess −1.1.

An uncomplicated left hemicolectomy is performed and the patient is sent from the recovery area back to a general surgical ward, having been cardiovascularly stable and maintaining his oxygen saturation at 94% on air. Analgesia using a patient-controlled analgesia (PCA) system has been established using morphine with a background infusion of 3 mg/h running. You are asked to see him 5 h postoperatively because he has become drowsy and his respiratory rate is less than 6 breaths/min. Arterial blood gases on air now show pH 7.30; $Paco_2$ 7.1 kPa; Pao_2 5.4 kPa; HCO_3^- 26 mmol; base excess −4.2.

Questions

1. Define the types of respiratory failure and comment on the pre- and postoperative blood-gas results.
2. Outline briefly the possible causes of inadequate ventilation in this patient. How would you treat him?
3. What devices are available for supplying supplementary oxygen to a patient on the ward?
4. If the patient remains drowsy and confused and a repeat set of arterial blood gases show pH 7.21; $Paco_2$ 6.6; Pao_2 6.0 kPa; HCO_3^- 20; base excess −6.1 on 60% inspired oxygen and a chest X-ray shows increased right middle and lower zone shadowing, what would be your course of action?
5. What are the normal ventilator settings? What is PEEP?
6. Briefly discuss weaning the patient from a ventilator.

Answers

1. Respiratory failure occurs when there is an inability to produce effective gas exchange such that the oxygen tension in blood falls while that of carbon dioxide rises. Respiratory failure is said to be present in a patient at rest, breathing air at 101.3 kPa pressure (1 atm), if the arterial Pa_{O_2} is <8 kPa and/or the Pa_{CO_2} is >6.7 kPa. It may be acute or chronic in nature.
   Chronic respiratory failure has been divided into:
   (a) Type I: low Pa_{O_2} with normal or slightly reduced Pa_{CO_2}.
   (b) Type II: low Pa_{O_2} with elevated Pa_{CO_2}.
   Chronic respiratory failure is distinguished from acute respiratory failure by the presence of renal compensation seen on blood-gas analysis.
   In the example given there is no evidence of respiratory failure and a Pa_{O_2} of 10.1 kPa in a 74-year-old man with mild COAD is not unexpected. With increasing age there is a gradual fall in resting Pa_{CO_2}.
   The postoperative arterial blood gases show respiratory failure to be present and a respiratory acidosis.
2. Respiratory inadequacy may be due to one factor or a combination of factors from the following list:
   (a) Upper airway obstruction – oedema, tumour, tongue.
   (b) Lower airway obstruction – asthma, aspiration.
   (c) Central respiratory depression – drugs, hypoxia.
   (d) Respiratory muscle weakness – neuropathy, neuromuscular blocking drug.
   (e) Thoracic cage abnormality – injury, kyphoscoliosis.
   (f) Diaphragmatic problem – mechanical splinting (obesity, abdominal distension).
   (g) Lung and pleural space pathology – COAD, inhalational injury, pneumothorax.
   There is a spectrum of treatments ranging from a simple jaw thrust (to relieve obstruction by the tongue) to mechanical ventilation, depending on the cause.
   In this case history there are several possible causes:
   (a) Central depression by the morphine (3 mg/h plus any bolus doses may be an overdose in a 74-year-old man) and subsequent hypoxia.
   (b) Diaphragmatic splinting (he is obese and a painful abdominal operation will tend to reduce abdominal wall movement).
   (c) COAD, and the possibility of aspiration having occurred.

Treatment will consist of oxygen supplementation via a facemask and encouraging the patient to take deep breaths. The PCA should be stopped. If the patient is too drowsy to comply, intravenous naloxone may be titrated to improve respiratory effort. The chest should be ausculated and a chest X-ray obtained if there are clinical signs of chest pathology. Respiratory rate and depth should be closely monitored, preferably in combination with oxygen saturation, measured using a pulse oximeter. Blood gases should be repeated to assess the effectiveness of your actions.

3. Oxygen therapy is an increase in the fraction of oxygen (F_{IO_2}) in the inspired gas (an increase in partial pressure). There are several ways to supply supplementary oxygen to a patient on a ward:
   (a) *Uncontrolled oxygen therapy*, e.g. via a Hudson mask. This is used routinely in the recovery room and also on general wards. It is suitable for the majority of patients, where the exact inspired oxygen concentration is not critical. The F_{IO_2} varies with the patient's respiratory rate and depth. The faster the respiratory rate, the less time for fresh gas to flush into the mask, and the more likely the patient is to rebreathe some of his own expired air and draw in room air. The concentration of oxygen is normally delivered around 40% but can be increased if a reservoir bag is added. Nasal cannulae perform a similar function to masks and some patients tolerate them better.
   (b) *Controlled oxygen therapy.* The Venturi masks (high-air-flow oxygen enrichment masks) entrain a fixed amount of room air as the oxygen is delivered, e.g. 2 l of oxygen can entrain around 48 l of air. Such large volumes ensure there is little change in the oxygen concentration of the mixture throughout the respiratory cycle. The inspired oxygen concentration is set for a particular Venturi mask.
   (c) *Continuous positive airway pressure (CPAP)* consists of a tight-fitting face or nasal mask and a high flow of oxygen-enriched air, such that there is a positive pressure in the mask, and therefore the airways, throughout the respiratory cycle. This prevents collapse of distal airway during expiration and helps improve gas exchange. The tight-fitting mask is unpleasant and many patients will not tolerate it.

4. The patient is not maintaining his oxygenation and the hypoxia will add to his confusion. Further intervention on the ward, such as CPAP, is unlikely to improve matters. The anaesthetist should be contacted as the patient may require urgent intubation and ventilation and arrangements for transfer to the intensive care unit should be made.

   The increased shadowing in the right lung may be due to collapse or consolidation or may represent aspiration of gastric contents.
5. Conventional ventilation is by intermittent positive-pressure ventilation (IPPV) via an endotracheal tube. In adults the rate is usually 10–12 breaths/min with tidal volumes of 10 ml/kg. The oxygen concentration is set to produce a satisfactory $Pa\text{O}_2$ on arterial blood-gas samples, generally >10 kPa depending on premorbid levels. Numerous modes of ventilation are available.

   PEEP Stands for positive end-expiratory pressure. The positive airway pressure at the end of expiration holds open the airways, helps reduce atelectasis and can improve gas exchange. It can be used as an addition to the other forms of ventilation. One must take care in its use as it may compromise cardiac output by reducing venous return.
6. Weaning is usually straightforward, but varies depending upon the reason for initial ventilation and on the duration of ventilation. Many criteria have been suggested for use in identifying when weaning can commence, such as:
   (a) Resolution of the condition leading to ventilation.
   (b) Absence of major organ failure.
   (c) Absence of fever or major infection.
   (d) No severe metabolic derangement.
   (e) Good nutritional state.
   (f) Improving respiratory function.

   The $Fi\text{O}_2$ should be less than 0.6 (i.e. <60% oxygen). As the patient's spontaneous rate increases, so the rate of breaths delivered by the ventilator is reduced. The breaths delivered by the ventilator can be synchronized with the spontaneous breaths (spontaneous intermittent mandatory ventilation mode), which is more acceptable to the patient. Eventually the patient, although still intubated, is performing all the breaths, at which stage he can be placed on a T-piece. This consists of tubing through which oxygen-enriched air is passed, with an expiratory limb about 30 cm long to prevent entrainment of room air. Additional support can be given by the addition of a pressure valve on the expiratory limb so that the patient receives CPAP. When the patient is able to maintain adequate arterial blood gases on the T-piece, he may be extubated and placed on a simple facemask.

Mark Smith
Alastair Skelly

Case 24 Diagnostic laparoscopy: Acute abdomen

An 18-year-old woman presented to the casualty department with a 5-day history of increasing right iliac fossa and suprapubic pain. The pain was associated with fever and sweating. On examination there was tenderness and guarding in the lower abdomen. Rectal examination demonstrated right-sided tenderness.

Questions

1. What is your differential diagnosis?
2. What investigations would you perform?
3. In what emergency situations is diagnostic laparoscopy helpful?
4. What methods are there for the establishment of a pneumoperitoneum?
5. If the diagnostic laparoscopy was normal but the appendix was not seen, how would you proceed?
6. How would you close the port sites and why?

Answers

1. The causes of an acute abdomen in a young woman are numerous and may be classified as surgical, medical or gynaecological. The important question is whether or not surgery is indicated. Common causes include acute appendicitis, ectopic pregnancy, pelvic inflammatory disease, urinary tract infection, infective colitis, inflammatory bowel disease, ovarian cysts and torsion of an ovary. In a large proportion of cases, no cause for the pain will be found, in which case the term non-specific abdominal pain is applied.
2. As in all cases, investigations should be guided by the history. However, given the vague nature of the presentation it is vital that important diagnoses be ruled out. A pregnancy test should be performed on all women of child-bearing age. The urine should be tested for the presence of protein and

sent for microscopy, culture and sensitivity. If diarrhoea is a presenting symptom, a stool sample should also be taken. If there is a history of vaginal discharge, a high vaginal swab may reveal a sexually transmitted cause such as chlamydial infection. Baseline blood tests should include a full blood count, electrolytes and urea and plasma glucose. Imaging should be by abdominal ultrasound and a plain abdominal X-ray, if indicated. If the diagnosis is still uncertain and the clinical picture is suggestive of a surgical condition, diagnostic laparoscopy is the next investigation of choice.

3. Emergency diagnostic laparoscopy may be particularly useful in patients with acute abdominal pain in whom the decision to operate is in doubt. The case for this approach is strengthened by the fact that an increasing number of acute surgical conditions, such as appendicitis, acute cholecystitis, perforated duodenal ulcer, small-bowel obstruction due to adhesions, ectopic pregnancy and torsion of an ovary may all be diagnosed and managed laparoscopically.

   Laparoscopy may also aid the diagnosis of blunt trauma and penetrating injuries. However, patients in shock with obvious abdominal injury should have a laparotomy without delay. The same applies to those who on examination show signs of peritonitis, gross gastrointestinal blood loss or rectal or vaginal disruption.

   The kinds of injury to be expected from blunt trauma relate to the applied force, its direction, the presence of supporting structures and physical characteristics of the affected organs. Diagnostic laparoscopy for blunt trauma may be indicated where diagnostic peritoneal lavage or computed tomography (CT) scan findings are equivocal, for haemostasis of minor hepatic or splenic injuries, or for the evaluation of possible diaphragmatic injury.

   With penetrating trauma, those with obvious entry into the abdomen from a gunshot wound should undergo exploratory laparotomy. Patients sustaining high-velocity wounds should also have abdominal exploration regardless of evidence of abdominal penetration because shock waves may cause intraperitoneal injury without actually penetrating the peritoneum. Some abdominal gunshot wounds, especially if tangential, may have a low probability of entering the peritoneal cavity. In this case, and in stab wounds where the tract can be clearly visualized and does not breach the peritoneum, local wound exploration may be all that is necessary. It is important to note that the retroperitoneal organs are separate from the rest of the abdomen and may be injured without peritoneal signs, leading to a delay in diagnosis.

4. A pneumoperitoneum may be introduced using the open or closed technique. The open technique involves a direct cut-down on to the peritoneum through an infra- or supraumbilical incision. A pursestring suture is placed around the fascia of the incised linea alba and peritoneum to prevent excessive gas leakage when the port has been inserted. Alternatively a Hasson's port may be employed, in which case two strong nylon sutures are inserted on each side of the incision rather than a pursestring suture. The edges of both the linea alba and the peritoneum are incorporated in the suture which is pulled up, while at the same time inserting the external winged section of the port firmly into the opening in the peritoneal cavity, and the sutures locked into place. The inner port can then be advanced through the external port and firmly screwed into place.

   For the closed technique, after palpation of the abdomen to exclude a full bladder, a Veres needle is inserted. This spring-loaded device has an internal obturator which pushes back as the needle traverse the abdominal wall, and springs forward once the peritoneal cavity has been entered. The commonest site for insertion of the Veres needle is through a supra- or infraumbilical incision at an angle towards the patient's pelvis over the pelvic brim with the patient in the Trendelenburg position and the anterior abdominal wall raised by the surgeon's left hand.

   Confirmation that the Veres needle is in the peritoneal cavity may be gained by:

   (a) The audible hiss heard as air is drawn into the peritoneal cavity.
   (b) The falling meniscus of a drop of water placed on the hub of the Veress needle before insertion.
   (c) The inability to aspirate from the needle previously injected fluid.
   (d) The low initial insufflation pressure (less than 10 mmHg at 1 l/min).

   The open system of establishing pneumoperitoneum has been shown to be safer, faster and cheaper than the closed method. It is also particularly appropriate for use in patients who have had previous abdominal surgery where there is a possibility of underlying adhesions. Percutaneous ultrasonography has been used to identify adhesions between viscera and the anterior abdominal wall by noting the absence of motion during respiration.

5. If no cause for the abdominal pain is seen at diagnostic laparoscopy, it is imperative that the appendix is visualized. Every attempt should be made to do this laparoscopically. If this proves too difficult, the procedure should be converted to laparotomy by enlarging the right lower abdominal port site as an inflamed retrocaecal appendix could be missed laparoscopically. If on inspection the appendix seems normal, it is debatable whether it should be removed. The appendix may indeed be normal but it is also possible that serosal involvement may be minimal.
6. Incisional hernia following laparoscopy is reported as occurring after approximately 0.1% of diagnostic laparoscopies, and 0.25–1% of laparoscopic cholecystectomies. The vast majority occur in ports measuring 10 mm or more and are commonly located at the umbilicus. As these may become incarcerated, it is important to prevent this complication by suturing all port sites measuring 10 mm or more in layers. Smaller port sites are unlikely to result in incision hernia and may be closed with one or two interrupted sutures or adhesive tape.

Further reading

Bellem RV and Rudomanski J. (1993) Techniques of pneumoperitoneum. *Surgery Laparoscopy and Endoscopy* **3:** 42–3

Milkins RC and Wedgewood KR. (1994) Incisional hernia following laparoscopic surgery. *Minimally Invasive Therapy* **3:** 35–38

Paterson-Brown S and Garden J. (eds) (1994) *Principles and Practice of Surgical Laparoscopy.* WB Saunders, London

Charles C. Nduka
A.W. Darzi

Case 25 Management of postoperative electrolytes

A 76-year-old man presented with an incarcerated inguinal hernia. The hernia had been present for some years but he had several episodes of pain and was eager to have the hernia repaired.

He had a past medical history of mild hypertension and several episodes described as heart failure, for which he was on long-term diuretics. He smoked 20 cigarettes a day and admitted to 2 pints of beer each evening.

On examination he was a thin frail man weighing about 51 kg. He appeared debilitated and had obviously lost weight. His tongue was dry and he had poor skin turgor. Investigations done at this time showed Na 136 mmol/l; K 4.0 mmol/l; HCO_3^- 25 mmol/l; urea 8.0 mmol/l; creatinine 105 mmol/l.

He was admitted for surgery. On assessment it was thought that he was clinically dry and was given 2 l of 5% dextrose in the ward preoperatively. He had an uneventful operation with minimal blood loss. Intraoperatively he was given 1 l of Hartman's solution. Postoperatively the drip was left *in situ* with 1 l of 5% dextrose to run over 12 h. On returning to the ward he was noted to have poor urine output and the drip was speeded up, to run over 6 h. A further 2 l of 5% dextrose was written up to run 6-hourly as he was deemed to be dry.

The following day the patient was reluctant to take fluids orally and, although the urine output was much improved, the drip was left in place and he was written up for 1 l of dextrose saline 8-hourly.

On the second night the patient became agitated, confused and disoriented. In view of his alcohol history a provisional diagnosis of delirium tremens was made and he was commenced on intravenous heminevrin, running concurrently with his intravenous fluids. He settled.

The following day he was barely rousable and he was noted to have laboured breathing. The heminevrin was stopped but he failed to wake, although he did respond to pain. A diagnosis of aspiration pneumonia was made and he was transferred to the intensive therapy unit (ITU).

In ITU the electrolytes were measured and found to be Na 122 mmol/l; K 3.5 mmol/l; urea 5 mmol/l; creatinine 60 mmol/l.

Questions

1. What is the problem?
2. How did it happen?
3. How do we manage the problem?

Answers

1. This is a classic and unfortunately common example of iatrogenic electrolyte problems. He has normovolaemic hyponatraemia. This patient is suffering from the consequences of water overload and intoxication.
2. It is likely that this patient, while appearing dry and on diuretics, had no real reason for being grossly dehydrated and probably was normovolaemic. His initial electrolytes were normal and his urea and creatinine, at the upper-normal range, may reflect some impairment of renal function rather than dehydration. The 2 l of 5% dextrose preoperatively probably did no harm but he went to theatre normovolaemic with a water load.

   Intraoperatively he received a further litre of fluid. He is only 51 kg and he has now had 3 l of fluid, although intraoperative blood loss is likely to be negligible. Postoperatively he will have a stress response, albeit minor, after such a hernia repair. With antidiuretic hormone (ADH) and aldosterone secretion there will be a tendency to retain salt and water.

   Postoperatively his urine output was poor. This probably would have improved and observation would have been better than embarking on a 3 l/day regimen. It is highly unlikely that a 52-kg man who is already 3 l or more positive will require 3 l/day. The fluid chosen was 5% dextrose. In patients with a history of heart failure there is a fear of salt-containing solutions. If urine output was the problem then intravascular expansion is required and, of the fluids available, 5% dextrose is the least effective for that purpose.

   The problem of water overload is now established.

   Excretion of this water load necessitates the loss of salt and water. The ADH secretion compounds this problem and so the diuresis expected is not always seen. This is not inappropriate ADH as it is part of the normal response to surgery but it is inappropriate in the context of the patient becoming hypotonic.

When the patient was reluctant to take fluid orally, this may reflect the start of a confusional state. The urine output was adequate and would have been very dilute. Intravenous fluids in the form of dextrose saline were given – again 3 l/day. Dextrose saline does contain some salt but for every litre of dextrose saline there is 800 ml of free water. It is not a means of giving sodium, rather it is a slow way of giving water. The net effect unless the patient can produce a very dilute urine is the loss of some sodium and the retention of more water.

On the second night the patient became confused as hyponatraemia became a major problem. Alcohol was incorrectly invoked as the cause and the treatment was heminevrin. This often requires large volumes initially and this is again free water, accentuating the problem of hypotonic normovolaemic hyponatraemia.

The patient deteriorated either due to aspiration caused by reduced hyponatraemia or heminevrin or both or alternatively had a hypostatic problem with secretions because of a reduce level of consciousness.

3. The respiratory system needs to be managed to prevent hypoxia or further aspiration. The problem with the electrolytes is water overload. The patient is not salt-depleted or hypovolaemic. Aggressive fluid restriction will allow the patient to excrete the water. Fluids given should be isotonic saline with no free water. Occasionally the process can be accelerated by giving diuretics to increase rate of water loss.

In extreme circumstances there may be a case for using hypertonic saline but this is hazardous. First, it involves intravascular volume expansion and second, it may correct the problem too fast. The problem is neither volume depletion nor sodium deficit, so giving intravenous fluids and sodium is not appropriate.

The lessons are:

(a) Patients should be well-hydrated before surgery with full intravascular compartments but giving excess water may not be helpful.
(b) Postoperative reduced urinary output is not always fluid depletion.

(c) If intravascular volume replacement is necessary then it is best done using fluids which fill the space efficiently, such as colloids or salt solutions.
(d) Fluids of 3 l/day may be too much for small patients with small requirements.
(e) Dextrose saline is water with a bit of salt, not a balanced salt solution.
(f) All confusion is not delirium tremens. Heminevrin is in water and aggravates the problem. It is always given in parallel with intravenous fluids and often large volumes are given.

Further reading

Cohen R. (1991) Roles of the liver and kidney in acid–base regulation and its disorders. *British Journal of Anaesthesia* **67:** 154–164

Hawker R (1982) *Notebook of Medical Physiology, Renal and Body Fluids*, Churchill Livingstone, Edinburgh

Mayne P. (1994) *Clinical Chemistry in Diagnosis and Treatment*, 6th edn. Edward Arnold, London

Oh M and Carroll H. (1992) Disorders of sodium metabolism: hypernatraemia and hyponatraemia. *Critical Care Medicine* **9:** 630–632

Neil Soni
Geoffrey Raine

Case 26 Principles of local anaesthesia

A 30-year-old man presents in the clinic with a 6-month history of intermittent left inguinal swelling which was initially painless and easily reducible. Over the last week the swelling has become more painful and increasingly difficult to reduce. Past medical history include chronic backache due to a prolapsed disc. He has no history of allergy, but family history reveals that an older brother had died 'under anaesthesia' several years earlier. On account of this he specifically refuses to have a general anaesthetic if surgery is necessary.

Questions

1. What is the likely diagnosis?
2. In view of his refusal to have a general anaesthetic, what type of anaesthesia could be provided to enable surgery to be carried out?
3. Briefly describe the classification of local anaesthetic drugs commonly available, giving at least one example of each and the dosage required.
4. What are the contraindications, complications and possible risks in the use of these drugs?
5. What equipment would you require to carry out suitable local anaesthesia on this patient?
6. Describe the technical procedure for producing suitable local anaesthesia for this patient. What precautions would you take?

Answers

1. The likely diagnosis is that of a left inguinal hernia. The hernia may be either a direct one or an indirect one. The problem should be investigated by taking a full history and detailed clinical examination. In this patient, who possibly has a family history associated with an anaesthetic death, a very detailed family history is indicated.
2. Local or regional anaesthesia could be provided. In this particular situation, local infiltration may be all that is required.

This minimizes the number and type of drugs that may be used. The awake patient is able to notify the surgeon of any adverse symptoms following the administration of any drugs.

3. Local anaesthetics are classified under two groups:
   (a) Esters, e.g. cocaine and procaine.
   (b) Amides, e.g. lignocaine, prilocaine and bupivacaine.

   Cocaine is usually used topically in nasal mucosal anaesthesia and in concentrations of 4–10%, maximum dose 1–1.5 mg/kg. It is also a vasoconstrictor.

   Lignocaine is used either plain or with adrenaline. Used plain, the dosage is 2–3 mg/kg body weight with a maximum dosage of 200 mg. Used with adrenaline, the dosage is 4–7 mg/kg body weight up to a maximum of 500 mg. Lignocaine 1% has 10 mg lignocaine per millilitre; 2% lignocaine has 20 mg/ml. The maximum dose is therefore approximately 30 ml of 1% lignocaine (plain) for a 70 kg man.

   Bupivacaine (Marcain) is also presented either plain or with adrenaline. The dosage is 1–2 mg/kg body weight with a maximum dosage of 160 mg in 4 h. Bupivacaine 0.5% has 5 mg/ml and therefore the maximum dose is approximately 30 ml for an average 70-kg man.

4. Contraindications include:
   (a) Known hypersensitivity to anaesthetics or compounds of ester or amide type, or hypersensitivity to the preservatives and/or stabilizing agents, e.g. sodium metabisulphite and disodium edetate.
   (b) Use of local anaesthetics containing vasoconstrictors for anaesthesia of fingers, toes, tip of nose, ears and penis, as vasospasm may lead to distal gangrene.

   Bupivacaine is contraindicated for intravenous regional anaesthesia due to cardiotoxicity. Solutions containing adrenaline are contraindicated in patients with thyrotoxicosis, or severe heart disease, especially when tachycardia is already present.

   Complications and risks include intravascular injection, which may lead to toxicity with central nervous system symptoms and cardiovascular collapse.

   Neuritis, due to direct puncture of the neurolemma, may occur during injection. This is more common when the injection is near an articular area, e.g. ulnar nerve block at the groove on the medial condyle, peroneal block at the head of fibula.

5. Equipment required consists of a short-bevel, non-cutting needle, two sterile needles (one 18 G and one 25 G). The required local anaesthetic agent in the appropriate concentration is provided in a sterile pack. A sterile procedure pack along with an antiseptic cleaning fluid will be required. Trained assistance is also needed. Full resuscitation facilities should be available. Intravenous access must also be provided by means of at least a 16 G cannula before the local anaesthetic procedure is commenced.
6. The procedure is explained to the patient and the skin is cleaned and draped. The landmarks are identified – the anterior superior iliac spine and the pubic tubercle. A wheal is raised at a point on the skin of the anterior abdominal wall (2–3 cm superomedial to the junction of the medial and middle third of the inguinal ligament) by injecting 1–2 ml of a local anaesthetic agent. The local anaesthetic agent (e.g. 0.5% bupivacaine 8–12 ml) is then injected in a fan-like spread from this wheal in a subcutaneous plane. A needle is passed vertically downwards 1 cm medial to the anterior superior iliac spine until the fascia is pierced. Local anaesthetic 6–10 ml is injected (after aspiration to ensure that the needle is not in a blood vessel) to ensure that the ilioinguinal and lateral cutaneous nerve of the upper thigh are blocked. It may be necessary to inject more into the fascial plane once the inguinal ligament is exposed.

   The precautions include:

   (a) Confirming consent from patient.
   (b) Drugs history (exclude anticoagulation).
   (c) Confirming relevant landmarks.
   (d) Cross-checking the concentration and expiry date of the drugs.
   (e) Ensuring asepsis.
   (f) Aspirating from the needle before injecting the local anaesthetic.
   (g) Allowing the local anaesthetic agent time to take effect.

F.D. Opeyemi Babatola
Alastair Skelly

Case 27 Haematemesis/sepsis syndrome

Female 78 years	Weight 56 kg
Reason for admission:	Haematemesis
Medical history of note:	Rheumatoid arthritis for the past 3 years on non-steroidal anti-inflammatory drugs (NSAIDs) Drinks 2 glasses of white wine a night Congestive cardiac failure on digoxin and diuretics
Progress:	Gastric ulcer found at surgery and oversewn During the surgery she was given 8 units of blood, 4 units of fresh frozen plasma and 6 units of platelets Antibiotics – cefuroxime and metronidazole Recovery from surgery was apparently uneventful She suddenly collapsed 24 h later – she was resuscitated and taken to the intensive therapy unit (ITU)
Admission to ITU:	Blood pressure 70/40 mmHg Pulse rate 126 beats/min and irregular Temperature 38.4°C Electrocardiogram (ECG) – atrial fibrillation plus depressed ST segments in augmented leads 1 and 2 chest leads V3–V6 Chest X-ray – right lower lobe consolidation and increased hilar shadowing Kerly B lines and diffuse opacification throughout the lung fields
Blood tests:	Haemoglobin 17.8 g/dl Packed cell volume 51 Platelets 150–400 $\times 10^9$/l White cell count 17.4 $\times 10^9$/l C-reactive protein 240 mg/l

Cardiac enzymes – normal
Na^+ 132 mmol/l
K^+ 5.9 mmol/l
Urea 28.9 mmol/l
Creatinine 190 μmol/l
pH 7.18
$P\text{CO}_2$ 7.8 kPa
$P\text{O}_2$ 6.8 kPa
BE −18.2 mmol/l
Saturation 84% on 60% oxygen
Central venous pressure 19 cmH_2O
Pulmonary arterial wedge pressure 26 mmHg
Cadiac output (CO) 3 litres/mm
Cardiac index 1.9 ml/min/m^2
Systemic vascular resistance index (SVRI) 600 dynes/cm^2
$V\text{O}_2$ 80 ml/min
$D\text{O}_2$ 420 ml/min

Questions

1. What is the most likely cause of her haematemesis? Give a brief discussion of the factors that will influence the incidence.
2. What was the probable cause of her initial collapse?
3. On admission to the ITU, what was the provisional diagnosis?
4. What are the clinical features of this diagnosis?
5. What is the pathophysiology of the diagnosis?
6. What are the principles of management?

Answers

1. Gastric ulcer related to NSAIDs. The incidence is increased when the NSAIDs are taken continuously rather than intermittently when necessary. The incidence is directly related to the dose and the age of the patient. Haematemesis will often present without any symptoms. Drugs like ranitidine (H_2-receptor antagonist), omeprazole (proton pump inhibitor) and misoprostol (prostglandin E_1 analogue) have been

added in an attempt to decrease the incidence of gastric ulceration and haematemesis. (*Drugs and Therapeutics Bulletin*, 1994).

It is most unlikely that the haematemesis would be caused by the alcohol intake.

2. Congestive cardiac failure (CCF) following excessive blood transfusion.
3. CCF with superimposed sepsis syndrome. It is important to exclude an acute myocardial infarction. The chest X-ray shows congestion of the lungs related to cardiac failure. There is also right lower lobe consolidation probably due to aspiration that most likely occurred prior or during the period of collapse and resuscitation.
4. The sepsis syndrome (systemic inflammatory response syndrome; SIRS) is a constellation of clinical findings that identifies an inflammatory process with systemic involvement (Ball and Bone, 1989).

   When SIRS is associated with an infectious process it is known as sepsis.

   The clinical features of this syndrome are:

   (a) Fever – body temperature greater than 38°C or hypothermia less than 36°C.
   (b) Heart rate greater than 90 beats/min.
   (c) Tachypnoea – respiratory rate greater than 20 breaths/min or hyperventilation indicated by a $P\text{CO}_2$ of less than 32 mmHg or a minute volume of greater than 10 l/min.
   (d) Alteration of the white cell count – leukocytosis (greater than 12 000 cells/mm) or leukopenia (less than 400 cells/mm) or a presence of 10% or more immature neutrophils.

   In severe sepsis, organ dysfunction occurs due mainly to hypoperfusion abnormalities (Marino, 1900; Landlow and Anderson, 1994):

   (a) Lactic acid greater than 2 mm/l.
   (b) Oliguria – urine production of less than 0.5 ml/kg per h.
   (c) $Pa\text{O}_2/F\text{iO}_2$ of less than 250.
   (d) Hypotension – systolic blood pressure of less than 90 mmHg or a drop in systolic blood pressure by more than 40 mmHg.
   (e) Altered mental state.
5. In response to:
   (a) Infection:
      (i) Endotoxin, which is the lipopolysaccharide contained in the cell wall of Gram-negative bacteria.

- (ii) Peptidoglycan precursors and other components of Gram-positive bacteria cell walls and exotoxins.
- (iii) Viruses.
- (iv) Fungi.

(b) Trauma.
(c) Haemorrhage.
(d) Blood.

Macrophages and circulating monocytes are stimulated to produce:

(e) Cytokines that are inflammatory proteins (Schlag *et al.*, 1993; Redl and Schlag, 1994).
(f) Nitric oxide – the inducible form is coded by chromosome 17 (Hillhouse, 1994; Vallance and Collier, 1994).

There is ample evidence to show that shock, for whatever reason, will result in splanchnic hypoperfusion. This leads to local gut ischaemia with resultant damage to the gut epithelium. This damaged epithelium will be unable to prevent translocation of bacteria from the gut into the blood stream.

These bacteria will then stimulate macrophages and monocytes (Fig. 27.1) to produce a whole host of inflammatory proteins known as cytokines. These cytokines will then stimulate the conversion of arginine to citrulline under the influence of nitric oxide synthases (NOS, which are large complex proteins) with the production of nitric oxide in large amounts. This nitric oxide will then stimulate the production of cyclic guanosine monophosphate (GMP) from guanosine triphosphate (Fig. 27.2).

In addition, platelets and the complement system are activated (Hoeft and Mann, 1994).

(a) *Tumor necrosis factor (TNF).* TNF-alpha, also known as cachectin, is one of the earliest and most important cytokines to be released. There is a direct correlation between the level of TNF-alpha and the degree of organ dysfunction.

TNF-alpha stimulates polymorphonucleocytes to degranulate either before or once they have attached to the endothelial cell membrane. A large number of cytotoxic substances are thus released, causing endothelial damage. This will then allow movement of fluid into the interstitial tissue.

TNF-alpha is one of the cytokines that stimulates nitric oxide production.

Infection
Trauma
Haemorrhage
Cardiac
Shock
Translocation of bacteria from the gut
Macrophages and monocytes
ITL-1
Nitric oxide
TNF-alpha
Complement
ITL-8 (NAP)
Clinical symptoms
Anaphylatoxins C3a/C5a/C5b-9
PMN
Hydrogen peroxide oxygen free radicles
ITL-6
Platelets
+
Tissue factor plasminogen activator
Damage to endothelium
Leaking capillaries
Localized microaggregates
Interstitial oedema
Hypoxaemia

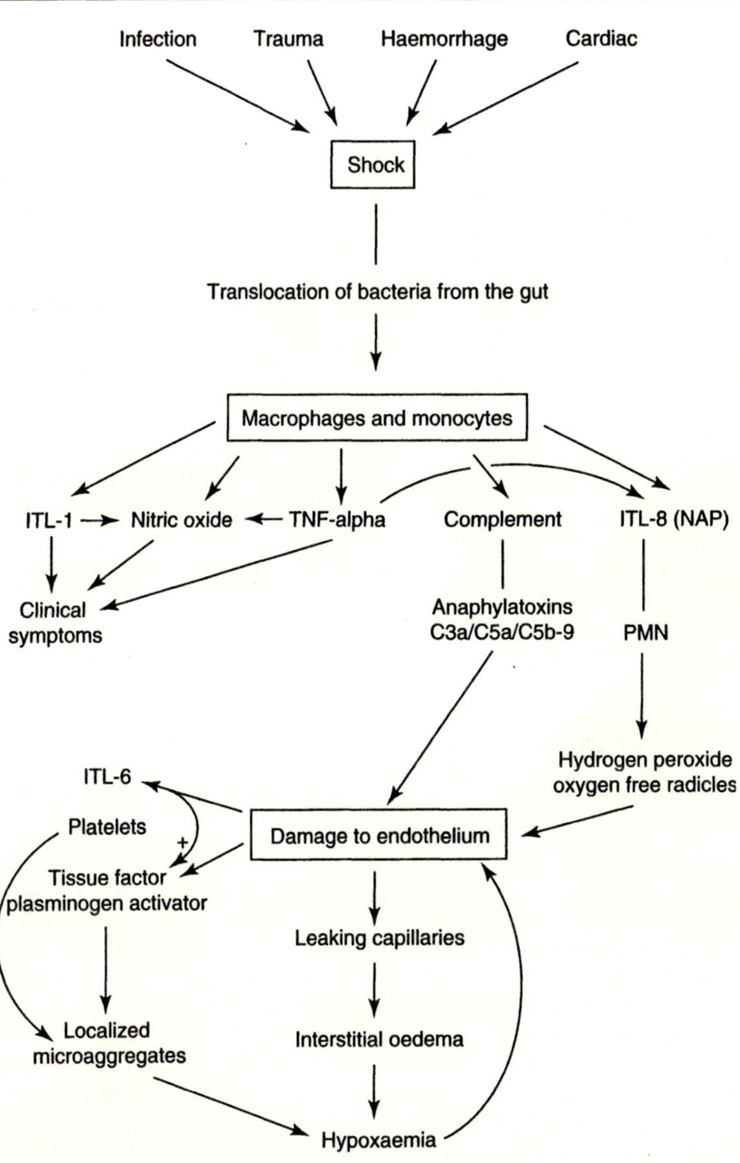

Fig. 27.1

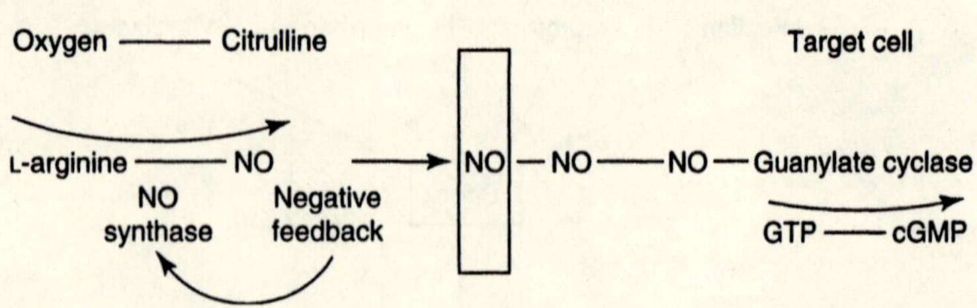

Fig. 27.2

TNF-alpha also helps to stimulate the activation of the complement system that results in the production of anaphylatoxins (i.e. C3a/C5a/C5b-9). This will result in further damage to the endothelium.

(b) *Interleukin-1.* This has a considerable structural and functional homology with TNF-alpha. It also stimulates the production of nitric oxide and is responsible for most of the clinical symptoms of the sepsis syndrome.

(c) *Interleukin-8.* This is also known as neutrophil-activating peptide (NAP-1). This is an important mediator as it forms a vital link between monocytes, macrophages and polymorphonuclear leukocytes.

The levels of interleukin-8 also closely correlate with the degree of organ dysfunction. As the name suggests, it attracts neutrophils to an area where they will then degranulate, resulting in the release of a number of toxic substances such as hydrogen peroxide and oxygen free radicals (Baxter, 1994). These substances will then cause localized damage, increased capillary permeability, interstitial oedema, hypoxaemia and further cell damage.

(d) *Interleukin-6.* Endothelial activation results in increased adhesion properties, with the secondary release of interleukin-6 and a subsequent procoagulant reaction. This will further stimulate those activated endothelial cells to produce tissue factor plasminogen activator, and show a decreased expression of thrombomodulin. Microaggregates with localized capillary obstruction then occur with subsequent further cell damage.

Clinically the above changes will manifest with progressive dysfunction in multiple organs, resulting in the multi-organ dysfunction syndrome.

(a) *Lung.* The capillary leakage will result in dense consolidation and alveolar haemorrhage, with hyaline membrane formation (ARDS = adult respiratory distress syndrome, better known as the acute respiratory distress syndrome).

(b) *Kidneys.* Systemic hypotension leads to decreased blood flow to the kidneys, resulting in renal artery constriction and renal medullary hypoxaemia. Endotoxin may itself cause damage directly to the tubules, as can a large number of drugs, e.g. Frusemide in high doses, cephalosporins and aminoglycosides. This leads to acute tubular necrosis.

(c) *Brain.* Metabolic abnormalities occur, resulting in the development of a septic encephlopathy. The metabolic abnormalities are probably the same ones that characterize the hepatic encephalopathy, i.e. there is an increase in aromatic amino acids which cross the blood–brain barrier where they are metabolized, with the resultant production of false neurotransmitters.

(d) *Liver.* Damage to the Kupffer cells as well as the hepatocytes occurs either directly or because of the decreased blood flow. One of the earliest signs is an increase in liver transaminases and intrahepatic cholestasis. Clinically this manifests with unexplained jaundice.

(e) *Heart.* The effect on the cardiovascular system is due to the production of nitric oxide in large amounts as well as the production of cardiac-inhibiting factors. The onset of myocardial dysfunction can occur within 2 h of onset of the inflammatory process. There is a depression of the cardiac myocyte with a resultant decrease in ejection fraction. This is thought to be due to the inhibition of the adenosine triphosphate-dependent calcium transport mechanism, resulting in a decreased movement of calcium into the cell as well as release from the sarcoplasmic reticulum.

The effect of the nitric oxide is to cause marked vasodilatation, which results in a drop in the diastolic blood pressure and the systemic vascular resistance.

(i) Early sepsis: low pulmonary capillary wedge pressure (PCWP), high CO, low systemic vascular resistance (SVR).
(ii) Late sepsis: high PCWP, normal CO, normal SVR.
(iii) Terminal sepsis: high PCWP, low CO, high SVR.

6. The management strategies are:
   (a) Restore the haemodynamic abnormalities by fluid therapy, vasodilators and inotropes.
   (b) Eradicate the infection. (In fewer than 50% of cases will a causative organism be found.)
   (c) Keep the oxygen consumption (Vo_2) high enough to match the hypermetabolic rate that occurs in sepsis – keep the lactic acid level below 2 mm/l.

References and further reading

See Case 2.

Charles Schamulian

Case 28 ATLS management in trauma

A 25-year-old woman is brought to your accident and emergency department following a road traffic accident. You are told that she crashed her car into the rear of a lorry. There was considerable deformation of the front of her car (front fender pushed back more than 25 cm). She was not wearing a seat belt. The steering wheel was damaged and the front windscreen was cracked in a 'bullseye' pattern and blood-stained. She was noted to be unresponsive and shocked. The paramedics proceeded as follows:

1. Applied a well-fitting neck brace.
2. Inserted an oral airway of correct size.
3. Administered oxygen at 6 l/min via mask device.
4. Following extrication she was placed on a long spine board and moved to your hospital.
5. Journey time reported as 15 min.
6. On arrival she is taken to resuscitation area. You are present and in charge of the hospital's trauma team. Your team works to Advanced Trauma Life Support (ATLS) assessment and initial management guidelines.

Questions

1. Outline your overall management strategy and defend it!
2. Given the history and, in particular, the mechanism of injury, what life-threatening conditions would you look for in each element of the primary survey? How might you deal with these conditions and in what order?
3. There is strong evidence to suspect cervical spine injury in this patient. Describe your strategy for care of the cervical spine during your management. At what stage may it be cleared and the collar or brace removed?
4. This patient was described as being shocked by the paramedics but no detail was given. Define shock and discuss the various aetiologies and presentations.
5. In the secondary survey you will assess the abdomen and pelvis in detail. Describe your approach. Assuming a pelvic fracture is present, how will this influence your management?

6. Compare and contrast the role of computed tomography (CT) scanning and diagnostic peritoneal lavage (DPL) in patient management.

Answers

1. Trauma is a unique morbid condition characterized by urgency. Trauma kills and maims in reproducible time frames; for example, an obstructed airway will lead to irreversible brain injury and death in a matter of minutes and must clearly take precedence over ongoing blood loss. The ATLS system teaches an approach to trauma care that will identify the greatest threat or threats to life. The approach does not require you to establish a definitive diagnosis.

   Assuming a trained team is present, a horizontal approach is optimal. Members of the team synchronously assess and manage the airway (with cervical spine control), the breathing mechanism, the circulatory system and the neurological system. The ATLS system may also be utilized by one individual assessor, commencing with the airway and proceeding vertically down through breathing and circulation and so on. For descriptive purposes, the management strategy is best described using a vertical approach, although our team will, in practice, apply it horizontally.

   Management involves an initial assessment and resuscitation period, the elements of which are:
   (a) The primary survey.
   (b) The resuscitation phase.
   (c) The secondary survey.
   (d) Initiation of definitive care.

   As the purpose of the primary survey is to uncover life-threatening injuries, it follows that these injuries are managed as they are found. Therefore, the primary survey and resuscitation phase are concurrent. Once the patient has been fully stabilized, the individual or team may proceed to a full secondary survey. This consists of a head-to-toe examination of a fully undressed patient – an examination which must include the back. Most requisite investigations may be safely performed at this time. As trauma is a dynamic condition, all of these activities should be repeated frequently.

Any deterioration should direct the examiner back to the primary survey.

The primary survey is an ABC approach to assessment. It consists of the following processes:

A Airway assessment and maintenance while controlling the cervical spine.
B Breathing assessment and ventilation control.
C Circulatory assessment and haemorrhage control.
D Disability: assessment of neurological status.
E Exposure of the patient and control of the environment.

This approach allows identification and management, in appropriate order, of any life-threatening condition that may be present. It needs no further defence.

2. The mechanism of injury in this case is striking. An unrestrained driver involved in a head-on collision will have predictable injury patterns. The damage to the windscreen suggests a 'bullseye' impact, putting at risk the airway as a result of facial injury or fracture, and the cervical spine as a result of sudden flexion or extension. It is therefore safe practice to assume injury to the airway and neck and to take appropriate action. Note that in this case the paramedics immobilized the cervical spine and inserted an oral airway. Due to her conscious level (unresponsive) there is an urgent need for a definitive airway to ensure patency and allow adequate ventilation. The bent steering wheel and the front bumper deformation suggest considerable force applied to chest and abdomen. Forward motion sufficient to deform the steering wheel should also raise suspicion of injury to the pelvis and lower limbs resulting from impact on the dashboard and associated structures. Therefore, in assessing B of the ABCs, you should look for evidence of tension pneumothorax, massive haemothorax, cardiac tamponade, flail chest and pulmonary contusion and myocardial contusion. Each of these conditions needs to be sought, and if present, dealt with.

   Turning to the circulation, careful assessment of the abdomen for signs of intra-abdominal bleeding must take a high priority. Equally, the pelvis is at risk of disruptive injury, which is associated with severe and ongoing haemorrhage. Injury to lower limbs, often at multiple sites, should be suspected and may be sufficient to cause severe haemorrhagic shock. The impact of head and face on the windscreen may, in addition to putting the airway at risk, result in serious head injury which should be picked up during assessment of D.

Turning to management, each lesion should be dealt with in the order found. The airway must be secured with the cervical spine immobilized and high-flow oxygen (12 l/min) administered via a mask with reservoir bag. Life-threatening lesions in B are dealt with by needle thoracocentesis or tube thoracostomy or pericardial aspiration, depending on the lesion found. Flail chest with underlying contusion may mandate intubation and controlled ventilation. Cardiac injury requires the patient to be monitored and nursed in a cardiac intensive therapy unit. Circulation problems are treated with haemorrhage control (which may require operative intervention) and vigorous intravenous fluid therapy. Fracture of the pelvis may require the application of an external fixator to bring catastrophic haemorrhage under control. Life-threatening head injury requires early recognition, airway and ventilation control and early consultation with a neurosurgeon.

3. Care of the cervical spine in this case began at the roadside. In the hospital setting the cervical spine should be protected in one of two ways: either by manual in-line immobilization (note: not traction) or by the application of a well-fitting semirigid collar or brace coupled with sandbags placed either side of the neck and a broad adhesive tape placed across the forehead – in the jargon of ATLS, this is known as 'collar, sandbags and tape'!

   At some convenient stage, either during the primary survey or secondary survey, a cross-table lateral X-ray of the cervical spine is taken. All seven vertebrae and the upper border of T1 must be visible. The purpose of this film is not to clear the cervical spine and remove the collar; rather it is to draw attention to particular patterns of injury which will further reinforce spinal protection measures and prompt attending medical staff to seek expert help.

   Final clearance of the spine from injury is not the task of the initial assessment team. This is for experts to consider later. This means that most patients will leave the resuscitation room for ward, intensive care unit or theatre with the neck still immobilized. In practice, it may be many days and then only following further films or even CT, before immobilization devices are removed.

4. Shock is an abnormality of the circulatory system resulting in inadequate organ perfusion and tissue oxygenation. The most common aetiology following trauma is hypovolaemic shock due to blood loss (haemorrhagic shock), but there are other important causes. Non-haemorrhagic causes include cardiogenic shock, which is associated with injuries above the diaphragm and may coexist with haemorrhagic shock. A high index of suspicion and a knowledge of the mechanism of injury are important. Cardiogenic shock is a reflection of myocardial dysfunction and is usually seen following cardiac tamponade, myocardial contusion or, more rarely, following air embolism and myocardial infarction. Cardiac tamponade is most common after penetrating chest trauma, whereas myocardial contusion injury is associated with rapid deceleration blunt impact to the thorax. Other non-haemorrhagic causes include tension pneumothorax, septicaemic and neurogenic shock. Tension pneumothorax may mimic cardiac tamponade but the two are readily differentiated at initial clinical assessment in the primary survey – they may, of course, coexist. Spinal cord injury produces hypotension due to loss of sympathetic tone. Therefore, the classic picture of isolated neurogenic shock is hypotension without tachycardia; the patient is pink and warm and there is no narrowing of pulse pressure.

   Septicaemic shock is rare in the so-called golden hour of trauma. Typically, it follows penetrating abdominal injury where there is delay in initiating management – widespread faecal peritonitis supervenes and has a very high mortality. Patients with septic shock may be indistinguishable from those with the haemorrhagic variety. The history, the presence of delay and careful clinical assessment may help distinguish – remember, they are likely to coexist.

5. You may have had to survey the abdomen rapidly during the primary survey, perhaps as part of a hunt for a cause of obvious haemorrhagic shock. However, your secondary survey examination will be full and detailed. By this time the casualty will have had a *successfully* completed primary survey, the patient will be responding well to resuscitation efforts and there will be less of a sense of urgency. In addition, the patient will have been fully exposed (undressed) in

an appropriate environment – the E at the end of the primary survey. Examination now proceeds in conventional manner – inspection, percussion, palpation and auscultation, not forgetting perineal, rectal and vaginal assessment. A positive examination indicates the presence of intra-abdominal injury but a negative examination does not rule out injury and suggests the need for repeated assessments over time. The secondary survey is also the phase for 'fingers and tubes in orifices'. If clinically indicated, nasogastric and urinary catheters should be inserted, and blood and X-ray investigations initiated. It is also a convenient time to perform DPL (see below).

Significant fractures of the pelvis should have come to light during the primary survey – an X-ray of the pelvis is one of the three X-rays permitted during this phase. Fractures of the pelvis rarely occur in isolation. They are frequently associated with intra-abdominal injuries, retroperitoneal and pelvic vascular injury and haemorrhage from fractured pelvic bones. Major life-threatening haemorrhagic shock is a feature of these lesions. Massive volume replacement with careful monitoring may be called for. Continuing haemorrhage may require operative fixation – it is now appropriate to consider the application of pelvic external fixators in the resuscitation room.

6. DPL and CT both have a place in the management of the multiply injured patient. They are particularly indicated where abdominal examination following trauma is equivocal or where findings are obscured by, for example, fracture pelvis, spinal injury, loss of consciousness or alcohol. A further indication might be in a patient about to undergo prolonged investigation or anaesthesia for a lengthy non-abdominal procedure.

   DPL is very sensitive for intraperitoneal bleeding and can be done while resuscitation is proceeding. However, it is non-specific and may be overly sensitive; it is also an operative procedure ideally done by a trained surgeon. By contrast, CT is highly specific but requires a stable patient and cannot be performed in the resuscitation room. A complete CT examination must include the upper abdomen and pelvis and use both oral and intravenous contrast. CT is particularly useful for specific organs and for visualizing the retroperitoneum and pelvic structures.

Further reading

Advanced Trauma Life Support Program for Physicians, 5th edn (1993). ACS Publications, Chicago

Landon BA, Driscoll PA and Goodall JD. (1994) *An Atlas of Trauma Management – the First Hour.* Parthenon Publishing, London

Skinner D, Driscoll P and Earlam R. (eds) (1991) *ABC of Major Trauma.* British Medical Journal, London

James M. Ryan

Case 29 Smoking and the surgical patient

HW, a 62-year-old male, was referred by his general practitioner with an asymptomatic pulsatile abdominal swelling. He had been a heavy smoker (30 cigarettes a day) for the last 40 years and admitted to having a chronic cough with a clear expectorant. Clinical examination suggested the presence of an abdominal aortic aneurysm and an ultrasound scan confirmed a 6.5-cm infrarenal aneurysm, for which elective repair was recommended.

After appropriate preoperative assessment, the aneurysm was replaced with a tube graft and the patient was ventilated for 12 h prior to transfer to the ward. On the second postoperative day his recovery was complicated by the development of a mild pyrexia, confusion and tachypnoea. Investigation revealed collapse of the lower lobe of his left lung. Appropriate management was instituted and the patient subsequently recovered and was discharged from hospital on the 14th postoperative day.

Questions

1. Delineate the preoperative assessment of pulmonary risk factors in patients undergoing elective aortic surgery.
2. Briefly describe the effects of smoking on the respiratory and cardiovascular systems. How would these influence the preparation of patients for major elective surgery?
3. Describe the important operative and postoperative factors that increase the risk of developing pulmonary complications and any methods by which they can be minimized.
4. Outline the plan of management in a patient with postoperative atelectasis.

Answers

1. Patients undergoing vascular surgery are often elderly, with a high incidence of hypertension (40–60%), cardiac (50–70%) and lung disease (25–50%). Since the majority of patients on a vascular surgical ward are either current or ex-smokers, the risks of major pulmonary complications

following surgery are likely to be even higher than for all types of major abdominal surgery, when respiratory complications account for some 3–5% of deaths. However, adequate preoperative assessment and preparation, combined with suitable postoperative monitoring, can effectively reduce both the morbidity and mortality of major surgery.

Although it is difficult to quantify the risks of surgery for an individual patient, Pederson *et al.* (1986) have evaluated a series of preoperative factors which may help predict outcome. In decreasing order of importance they are:

(a) Clinical assessment: American Society of Anesthesiologists grade > 3.
(b) Cardiac failure.
(c) Cardiac risk index (Goldman).
(d) Pulmonary disease.
(e) Radiographic pulmonary abnormalities.
(f) Abnormal electrocardiogram (ECG).
(g) Emergency surgery.

(a) *Pulmonary disease*

The risk of developing postoperative pulmonary complications is higher in obese patients, those with chronic bronchitis and heavy smokers. Pre-existing pulmonary pathology may be highlighted by adequate preoperative assessment and investigations will include a chest radiograph. Although this is a poor indicator of functional impairment, patients with peripheral vascular disease have an increased risk of developing bronchogenic carcinoma because of their smoking and a chest X-ray should be examined to exclude this. Whilst other routine preoperative investigations may also provide indirect evidence of pulmonary insufficiency (ECG – right atrial or ventricular hypertrophy secondary to pulmonary hypertension; haematology – leukocytosis suggesting active lung infection; polycythaemia – chronic hypoxia), these changes are relatively non-specific.

In patients with chronic preoperative pulmonary symptoms, bacteriological examination of a sputum specimen should be performed and appropriate antibiotic therapy prescribed if cultures are positive. Finally, the functional assessment of pulmonary pathology requires spirometric studies which can be carried out at the bedside using portable equipment, such as the

PM2000 Personal Spirometer (Precision Medical Ltd.). Spirometry can effectively identify and quantify both obstructive (e.g. chronic bronchitis, asthma, emphysema) and restrictive (e.g. fibrosing alveolitis, sarcoidosis) pulmonary disease. The parameters measured include the vital capacity (V_c), forced expiratory volume in 1 s (FEV_1) and peak flow. V_c is reduced in both restrictive and obstructive lung disease. The FEV_1 is similarly affected, although the reduction is more marked in patients with airways obstruction and thus the FEV_1/V_c ratio remains normal in restrictive defects, whilst in airways obstruction the ratio is reduced below the predicted value. Measurement of peak flow on forced expiration is affected by the same factors as FEV_1 but provides a simple and rapid assessment of the severity of airways obstruction and can be used to monitor the effects of therapy.

Arterial blood-gas analysis is required if patients are dyspnoeic at rest or the results of spirometry are abnormal. A $Paco_2$ of >6.7 kPa indicates that elective postoperative ventilation will be required, since abdominal surgery may reduce functional residual capacity by some 50–60%, with this reduction persisting for up to 2 weeks.

The demonstration of significant pulmonary disease is not necessarily a contraindication to surgery but certainly identifies patients who will require additional postoperative care following their operation.

2. Smoking has a number of effects upon the cardiovascular and respiratory systems. In particular, the oxygen-carrying capacity of haemoglobin is reduced by the formation of carboxyhaemoglobin following inhalation of carbon monoxide, whilst nicotine produces tachycardia and hypertension by its effects on the sympathetic system and similarly increases coronary vascular resistance. These changes impair oxygen delivery to the myocardium, the requirements for which are increased by the tachycardia. Elimination of carboxyhaemoglobin with improvement in anginal symptoms occurs after 12–24 h abstention from smoking.

   Smoking also promotes the development of chronic bronchitis and augments the lung injury caused by other pulmonary irritants. The principal effects of smoking are to stimulate the hypersecretion of thick, viscid mucus and to impair tracheobronchial clearance. These factors increase the incidence of postoperative atelectasis and bronchopneumonia, particularly if the sputum is infected prior to surgery.

Recent reports indicate that smoking depresses the immune response by inducing a reduction in circulating immunoglobulin levels, natural killer cell activity, neutrophil chemotaxis and pulmonary alveolar macrophage activity. Full recovery of immune function occurs 6–8 weeks following cessation of smoking and this is associated with a significant reduction in the incidence of postoperative pulmonary complications.

In addition to a course of antibiotics for patients with infected sputum, preoperative chest physiotherapy, with percussion and postural drainage, together with humidified oxygen will facilitate clearance of secretions. Patients should also be instructed in deep-breathing exercises to improve the efficacy of diaphragmatic respiration, which will reduce the incidence of postoperative atelectasis. Bronchodilator therapy may also be required in patients with obstructive airway disease and this is usually continued throughout the perioperative period. Finally, if appropriate, weight reduction should be encouraged prior to surgery and patients should be strongly advised to stop smoking.

3. Following major abdominal surgery there is a change in the pattern of respiration from diaphragmatic to intercostal breathing which, together with abdominal distension resulting from postoperative ileus, increases the risk of pulmonary complications.

   In patients requiring replacement the infrarenal abdominal aorta surgery can be performed using either a transabdominal or retroperitoneal approach. It has been suggested that the latter is associated with better perioperative oxygenation and preservation of lung volume when compared to transabdominal exposure and may thus be safer in patients with significant pulmonary disease.

   Elective postoperative ventilation is required in grossly obese patients and in those in whom the vital capacity is <1 l. However, many anaesthetists choose electively to ventilate all patients undergoing aortic surgery, since this allows administration of adequate analgesia and time for rewarming. Excessive narcotic analgesia can result in postoperative hypoxemia and hypercapnia due to suppression of the ventilatory response to carbon dioxide and inhibition of coughing which impairs mucus clearance. The administration of narcotic analgesics can be reduced by infiltration of the wound with 0.25% bupivacaine, either at the time of closure or by continuous infusion via a catheter placed in the wound. Both of these methods, together with epidural anaesthesia used intra- and postoperatively, have been shown to reduce the incidence of respiratory complications, although the latter may limit early mobilization which also encourages deeper breathing.

Postoperative chest physiotherapy also reduces the incidence of pulmonary complications from some 48% to 22%. This, together with humidified oxygen and the selective use of bronchodilators, facilitates clearance of retain secretions. Similarly, instruction in deep breathing with a pillow supporting the abdominal wound is a simple but effective way of aiding sputum clearance. Occasionally bronchoscopy may be required, particularly when the secretions are viscid or there is radiological evidence of segmental lung collapse. In the event of respiratory failure ventilatory assistance may be necessary.

4. The commonest cause of postoperative respiratory compromise after abdominal surgery is atelectasis which presents with a mild pyrexia, tachypnoea, basilar rales and hypoxaemia with or without signs of basal consolidation. Atelectasis occurring within the first 24–48 h of surgery is usually the result of retained secretions. Postoperative fluid depletion and depression of the cough reflex predispose to development of bronchopneumonia, which is a well-recognized complication of atelectasis.

   The management of significant postoperative pulmonary complications includes:
   (a) Arterial blood-gas estimation.
   (b) Bedside spirometry.
   (c) Sputum culture.
   (d) Chest X-ray.

   Adequate pain control should be achieved to allow early mobilization and cooperation with the physiotherapist. Chest physiotherapy will include postural drainage, deep-breathing exercises and humidified oxygen delivered via a mechanical nebulizer to maintain a Pao_2 of >8 kPa. Some patients may also require oral or nasotracheal suction to remove secretions and stimulate coughing. Antibiotics should be prescribed based upon an initial Gram stain of a sputum specimen and changed depending upon the final bacteriological report and clinical progress.

In patients in whom a chest X-ray indicates lobar atelectasis with a significant reduction in lung volume, bronchoscopy and suction may be beneficial and ventilatory support will be required when either the P_{CO_2} is >6.5 kPa or the patient develops a significant respiratory acidosis (pH <7.31).

References and further reading

Barker AF. (1987) Respiratory complications. *Acute Medical Problems in the Postoperative Patient*, Porter GA (ed.). Churchill Livingstone, Edinburgh, pp. 83–105

Celli BR. (1993) Perioperative respiratory care of the patient undergoing upper abdominal surgery. *Clinics in Chest Medicine* **13:** 253–261

Ford GT, Rosenal TW, Clergue F and Whitelaw WA. (1993) Respiratory physiology in upper abdominal surgery. *Clinics in Chest Medicine* **14:** 237–252

Goldman L, Caldera DL, Nussbaum SR *et al.* (1977) Multifactorial index of cardiac risk in noncardiac surgical procedures. *New England Journal of Medicine* **297:** 845–850

Kiell CS and Ernst CB. (1993) Advances in management of abdominal aortic aneurysm. *Advances in Surgery* **26:** 73–98

Milledge JS. (1989) Preoperative assessment in patients with pre-existing disease of the respiratory system. In: *General Anaesthesia*, Nunn JF, Utting JE and Brown Jr BR (eds). Butterworth-Heinemann, Oxford, pp. 358–366

Pederson T, Eliasen K, Ravnborg M *et al.* (1986) Risk factors, complications and outcome in anaesthesia. A pilot study. *European Journal of Anaesthesia* **3:** 225–229

Smith G. (1992) Anaesthesia for Vascular Surgery. In: *Surgical Management of Vascular Disease*, Bell PRF, Jamieson CW and Ruckley CV (eds). WB Saunders, London, pp. 291–309

K.P. Kumar
M.J. Gough

Case 30 Benign prostatic hypertrophy

A 58-year-old male patient presented with a 2-year history of increasing nocturia, hesitancy of micturition and a poor intermittent stream. He had had one episode of proven lower urinary tract infection 18 months previously. He usually needed to pass urine two or three times at night. Daytime frequency was not a problem. The hesitancy was variable and worse at night. His urinary stream was slow, particularly in the morning. He denied any urgency, urinary incontinence, dysuria or haematuria. He was potent and had an active sex life. His general health was good apart from mild hypertension, for which he took a beta-blocker.

Questions

1. What is your preliminary diagnosis?
2. What would you expect to find on examination?
3. What investigations would you undertake?
4. What treatment would you advise?

Answers

1. The most likely diagnosis is bladder outflow obstruction due to prostatic enlargement. Statistically, it is much more likely that the enlargement is due to benign prostatic hypertrophy than to prostate carcinoma. With a relatively short history, bladder neck dyssynergia is not likely to be the underlying cause. The short history in the absence of any significant cause is not in favour of a urethral stricture.
2. The findings on examination are likely to be that his bladder is not palpably distended. Rectal examination reveals the size and consistency of the prostate and some attempt should be made to define whether the prostate is small, medium or large. The symmetry, surface and consistency of the gland should be assessed.
3. A urine sample should be taken for microscopy, culture and sensitivity. Renal function should be assessed with a measure of urea and electrolytes and a full blood count could be taken. To assess bladder outflow obstruction non-invasively,

the investigations of choice are an ultrasound residual urine volume estimation and a urinary flow rate. An ultrasound of the upper urinary tracts should also be included, to ensure that no upper urinary tract dilatation secondary to bladder outflow obstruction exists. Transrectal ultrasound of the prostate is not necessary unless there is a suspicion of malignancy, in which case biopsies may well be necessary if the prostate specific antigen level is raised. It is now becoming routine clinical practice to measure the prostate specific antigen level in all patients presenting with bladder outflow obstruction. A plain abdominal X-ray is probably unnecessary since bladder stones would be seen on ultrasound. An intravenous urogram is not a necessary part of the investigation of patients with bladder outflow obstruction unless there is a history of haematuria.

4. Treatment options will depend on the results of previous investigations. Patients who have significant symptoms of bladder outflow obstruction together with a residual urine volume of 100 ml or more and/or a significantly reduced urinary flow rate with a maximum flow of less than 15 ml/s and an average flow of 5 ml/s or less should be considered for active treatment. The standard advice would be that a transurethral resection of the prostate is the most likely surgical technique to provide relief of symptoms. This is a safe procedure, associated with a mortality of <0.1% but a re-operation rate of some 10%. The inevitable side-effect is retrograde ejaculation and all patients must be forewarned of this possibility.

   Patients with a less severe degree of bladder outflow obstruction, both symptomatically and objectively, could be offered an alternative form of treatment. Alpha-adrenergic blocking drugs relax the bladder neck and may improve the patient's symptoms, particularly those who have a small prostate in whom there is a significant degree of bladder outflow obstruction.

   The only alternative form of medical treatment is using a 5-alpha-reductase inhibitor which blocks the metabolism of testosterone to dihydrotestosterone. This brings about a shrinkage in the size of the prostate in some patients over a period of 6 months. Alpha-blockers are associated with postural hypotension. Approximately 5% of patients who take a 5-alpha-reductase inhibitor will experience either a reduction in libido or reduced potency.

Patients who are considered to be unfit for general or epidural anaesthesia may be considered for an intraprostatic stent or spiral. However, these are not to be recommended other than for short-term use and are associated with a significant failure rate. Balloon dilatation of the prostate has also been discarded as a satisfactory alternative to transurethral resection of the prostate, since the medium-term results have been disappointing. Thermotherapy and hyperthermia of the prostate by transurethral or transrectal devices have not been shown to be effective, other than in a minority of patients (20%) who present with a minor degree of bladder outflow obstruction.

The role of prostatic coagulation using laser energy is still under investigation. Early results show some promise, though patients experience retention following the treatment and therefore require postoperative catheterization. There is minimal blood loss but morbidity from urinary tract infections can be significant.

Further reading

Fair W and Weiss R. (1994) *Management of Prostate Diseases.* Professional Communications, New York

H.N. Whitfield

Case 31 Abdominal aortic aneurysm

A man aged 68 has an X-ray of his lumbar spine because of back pain and this is suggestive of an aortic aneurysm. Clinical examination and an ultrasound scan confirm the diagnosis and suggest that the aneurysm is 6 cm in diameter. The patient has had no previous medical problems but on direct questioning admits to mild angina on effort. His blood pressure is 170/90 mmHg and there are easily palpable pulses throughout both legs. There is a close relative with an aneurysm.

Questions

1. What is the likely pathological cause?
2. How would you plan further investigations for this patient?
3. What are the treatment options if the renal arteries are not involved?
4. What are the risks of intervention versus conservative management?

Answers

1. The most likely cause of the abdominal aneurysm in this patient is that this is a so-called atherosclerotic aneurysm. Other rarer causes of aneurysm, such as Marfan's syndrome, Ehlers–Danlos syndrome, Behçet's disease and syphilis, are less likely, especially in this age group. Another relatively uncommon cause of a rapidly enlarging and usually tender aneurysm is a primary infection of the aortic wall, with salmonella being the most commonly implicated organism. Such patients are usually pyrexial and often have positive blood cultures.

   The term atherosclerotic aneurysm is a poor one since epidemiologically these patients differ somewhat from patients with atherosclerotic occlusive disease (they tend to be younger with a greater male preponderance), suggesting that other factors must also be involved in their pathogenesis. It is thought that acquired risk factors such as smoking and hypertension in addition require an underlying genetic tendency to weakness of the aortic wall for aneurysmal degeneration to occur with increasing age.

Evidence of a genetic predisposition is also provided by the finding that there is an increased prevalence in first-degree relatives of affected patients. Recently it has been suggested that this genetic tendency may be due to defects or variants in type III collagen or in the production of enzymes such as elastase or metalloproteinases which may result in degradation of the aortic wall. To date it has not been possible to define the precise genes which are responsible, although this information may emerge in the future.

Some 5–10% of atherosclerotic aneurysms are complicated by surrounding inflammation, making surgery more difficult. These inflammatory aneurysms are thought to be due to an autoimmune reaction to lipid components of the aortic wall and in extreme cases can produce a syndrome similar to retroperitoneal fibrosis, with ureteric obstruction. Replacement of the aneurysm leads to a resolution of the inflammation.

2. Further investigations need to be addressed, first towards obtaining further information about the anatomy of the aneurysm and second, about the patient's risk for surgical intervention.
   (a) *Assessment of the aneurysm.* Ultrasound is the best screening test for abdominal aneurysms and provides a reliable and cost-effective method of follow-up in patients with known aneurysms. Ultrasound does not, however, reliably provide information about the level of the renal arteries in relation to the neck of the aneurysm and is not good at excluding a suprarenal or thoraco-abdominal component to the aneurysm. For this reason most surgeons prefer to have a computed tomography (CT) scan performed preoperatively. In addition CT will show if there is evidence of an inflammatory component to the aneurysm which appears as enhancing thickening outside the subintimal calcification in the aneurysm wall. CT may also show evidence of leak or contained rupture. Standard angiography is indicated where there is coexistent occlusive disease. The full extent of the aneurysm will not normally be revealed because the sac will contain thrombus and only the lumen size will be seen on angiography.

Magnetic resonance imaging and magnetic resonance angiography, where available, may also provide additional information. With the emergence of interest in endoluminal repair of aneurysm, the role of imaging has become particularly important, with spiral CT and computer reconstruction being used to assess the suitability of aneurysms for stenting.

(b) *Assessment for risk for surgery.* The principal risks to be assessed are those of cardiac, respiratory or renal dysfunction. Of these, cardiac disease is the most common cause of perioperative mortality following aneurysm repair. A careful history, with attention to details of exercise tolerance, combined with physical examination and chest X-ray, electrocardiogram (ECG) and simple blood tests should be performed on all patients. Respiratory function tests may be helpful in patients with dyspnoea or poor exercise tolerance, as may baseline blood-gas analysis. Routine stress ECG testing has high false-positive and negative rates and many patients will not tolerate the test because of claudication or breathlessness. Measurement of ejection fraction is useful and ejection fractions of 35% or less are a major risk factor for perioperative myocardial infarction. Similarly, stress echocardiography may also be of value, as may thallium-dipyridamole scanning. Patients thought to be at high cardiac risk may benefit from coronary angiography with a view to angioplasty or coronary bypass prior to their aneurysm repair.

3. The treatment options are either to manage the patient conservatively or to intervene. Symptoms such as abdominal or back pain increase the need for intervention and most symptomatic aneurysms should be operated on.

Intervention has traditionally been by open aneurysm repair. Midline or transverse abdominal incisions may be used and some surgeons favour an extraperitoneal approach. The neck of the aneurysm can then be clamped below the renal arteries and either a straight or bifurcated graft sewn in using the inlay technique. After the anastomoses have been successfully completed the aneurysm sac is sutured over the graft to cover it and to reduce the risk of subsequent fistulization to bowel. A bifurcated graft may be used to the iliac arteries if these are also diseased or taken down to the femoral arteries in the groins if there is associated occlusive disease.

More recently, the option of less invasive radiological techniques for treating abdominal aneurysm has been developed. Currently, however, only a relatively small number of centres are using these techniques and only on highly selected patients. In essence the technique involves inserting a graft through the femoral artery, passing it up into position below the renal arteries and fixing by using an expanding metal stent. Techniques for inserting both straight and bifurcated grafts are being developed.

4. In broad terms the risk of conservative management relates to the risk of rupture of the aneurysm, which in turn relates principally to the aneurysm size. Aneurysms of less than 4 cm in maximum diameter have a negligible (approaching zero) annual rupture rate in reported series. Aneurysms of 4–5.9 cm have a rupture rate of about 6% per annum and factors such as the patient's age and other risk factors need to be considered before recommending surgery. Patients with aneurysms greater than 6 cm in size are usually advised to have surgery and untreated have a rupture rate of 15% per annum or greater depending on size. Rupture carries a community mortality of 90% and, in those who reach hospital, a hospital mortality of 50%.

   The risks of intervention are mainly related to the operative and perioperative period with most deaths being due to cardiac events. Other postoperative risks include bleeding, distal embolization, infection and deep venous thrombosis and pulmonary embolism. It seems that after successful aneurysm surgery patients have a life expectancy similar to that of an age-matched population (and considerably better than the life expectancy of patients with occlusive disease).

   Operative risk appears to vary considerably between centres, with the best results usually coming from specialized vascular units. Such units can expect to have operative and perioperative mortality rates less than 5% for elective infrarenal aortic aneurysm repair. Important factors in achieving such good results include the availability of experienced vascular anaesthetists and intensive care and high-dependence unit facilities.

Further reading

Greenhalgh RM and Mannick JA. (1990) *The Cause and Management of Aneurysms.* WB Saunders, Philadelphia

Eastcott HHG. (1993) *Arterial Surgery*, 3rd edn. Churchill Livingstone, Edinburgh

Bell PRF, Jamieson CW and Ruckley CV. (1992) WB Saunders, Philadelphia

Rutherford RB. (1984) *Vascular Surgery*, 2nd edn. WB Saunders, Philadelphia

Averil O. Mansfield
Gerard Stansby

Case 32 Immunology/HIV

A 35-year-old male was referred to accident and emergency with a 3-day history of severe proctalgia, tenesmus and a mucus discharge with blood-staining after defecation.

Questions

1. What is the differential diagnosis?

   Further enquiry reveals that the patient is human immunodeficiency virus (HIV)-positive and that infection was homosexually acquired.

2. What signs would you look for on *general* examination which would suggest that the patient could be immunocompromised?

   On examination you notice a flat, painless, indurated, purplish-brown lesion on the hard palate and a small anal fissure. The patient is unable to tolerate digital rectal examination.
   Special investigations
   Temperature = 37.5°C
   White cell count = $2.0 \times 10^9/l$
   Neutrophils = 0.6
   Haemoglobin = 11.4 g/dl
   Glc = 4.5 mmol/l
3. What is your interpretation of your clinical findings and the results of the special investigations?
4. What surgical procedure is required?
5. What laboratory specimens should be sent and which investigations should be requested?

Answers

1. The differential diagnosis includes:
   (a) *Traumatic*
      (i) Anal fissure.
      (ii) Trauma.

  (b) Vascular – haemorrhoids.
  (c) *Neoplastic*
    (i) Carcinoma.
    (ii) Leukaemia.
  (d) *Inflammatory*
    (i) Ulcerative colitis.
    (ii) Crohn's disease.
  (e) *Infective*
    (i) Bacteria, e.g. gonococcus, *Chlamydia*, *Mycobacterium*, lymphogranuloma venereum, actinomycosis.
    (ii) Viruses, e.g. herpes simplex, cytomegalovirus.

2. The following conditions are highly suggestive of an immunocompromised state, although none is pathognomonic of HIV infection.
  (a) Peripheral generalized lymphadenopathy (PGL) – lymph nodes less than 2 cm in diameter, bilaterally symmetrical, smooth, rubbery, mobile and non-tender.
  (b) Oral lesions
    (i) *Oral Candida:* most commonly seen as a white curd which can be scraped off an erythematous base.
    (ii) *Oral hairy leukoplakia.* Painless, white, raised, striated lesions usually on the lateral border of the tongue. Caused by the Epstein–Barr virus.
    (iii) *Kaposi's sarcoma.* These tumours are usually painless (unless superinfected), non-pruritic and vary in colour from red-brown to purple. On the palate or gum area they may be flat or raised.
  (c) Cutaneous lesions
    (i) Kaposi's sarcoma.
    (ii) Extensive seborrhoeic dermatitis.
    (iii) Scarring from multidermatomal varicella-zoster infection (shingles).
    (iv) Scars from intravenous drug use.
    (v) Molluscum contagiosum. This benign condition, caused by a poxvirus, is most commonly seen in children with normal immune systems where it is a self-limiting condition. In immunocompromised individuals the molluscum are firm, pearly, umbilicated papules which are commonly found in the beard area, neck and upper chest.

3. The palatal lesion is suggestive of Kaposi's sarcoma which, in a patient who is HIV-positive, is an acquired immunodeficiency syndrome (AIDS)-defining diagnosis. This implies

severe immunocompromise. The patient is also neutropenic, which renders him highly susceptible to disseminated bacterial and fungal infections. He is at great risk of severe, possibly fatal systemic sepsis and therefore his condition and any possible surgical interventions should be discussed with colleagues who are experienced in the management of HIV-positive individuals.

4. Examination under anaesthesia. An anal fissure does not account for all the symptoms.
5. (a) Microbiology – MCS and acid-fast bacilli (includes MAI).
   (b) Virology – cytomegalovirus, herpes simplex virus, human papillomavirus.
   (c) Histopathology.

   As the patient is both neutropenic and pyrexial, blood cultures for MCS and AAFBs should be sent, as should swabs for gonococcus (rectal, throat, urethral).

One week later the patient passed faecal material per urethram and on examination he was noted to have multiple discharging perineal fistulae. Cytomegalovirus and mycobacteria are the commonest causes of perineal fistulae in individuals infected with HIV. Repeated examinations under anaesthesia and multiple biopsies may be required to isolate the causative organisms. The identification of one organism does not exclude the presence of further organisms and failure to respond to appropriate treatment must prompt further investigation and specimens.

Further reading

Libman H and Witzburg RA. (1993) *HIV Infection. A Clinical Manual*, 2nd edn. Little, Brown, Boston

Nye KE and Parkin JM. (1994) *HIV and AIDS*. Bios Scientific Publishers, Oxford

Lynn Riddell

Case 33 Colorectal cancer

A 75-year-old retired male accountant presented to accident and emergency with a 24-h history of lower abdominal pain, distention and absolute constipation. He had noticed progressively worse constipation over the last 4 weeks and on direct questioning admitted to noticing occasional episodes of bright red blood on the paper after defecation, which he had attributed to haemorrhoids. On examination he was apyrexial and in discomfort. Abdominal examination revealed a distended abdomen with visible peristalsis. Bowel sounds were increased and there was a non-tender, mobile mass in his left iliac fossa. Digital examination per rectum was normal. Sigmoidoscopy was normal to 20 cm. Proctoscopy revealed minor haemorrhoids.

Questions

1. Discuss the differential diagnosis.
2. Discuss the preoperative investigations and management you would perform.
3. At laparotomy a tumour of the lower signoid is found. What surgical options are available?
4. What is the definition of a polyp? How are polyps classified?
5. What are the high-risk groups for colorectal cancer?

Answers

1. (a) *Left-sided obstructing carcinoma.* This is the most likely diagnosis. The history is insidious and the patient is in the appropriate age range.
   (b) *Diverticular disease.* Diverticular disease causing large-bowel obstruction is unusual. Complicated diverticular disease can cause chronic obstruction. However, the mass in this patient is not tender and diverticular masses usually are, owing to local peritonism. The history in diverticular disease is longer, often many years, and attacks of acute diverticulitis may have been experienced in the past. Loops of small bowel may

become adherent to the diverticular segment and become obstructed, resulting in acute small intestinal obstruction.

(c) *Volvulus.* The sigmoid colon is the most common part of the large intestine to undergo volvulus. It occurs in institutionalized, elderly and chronically constipated patients. The torted segment can become ischaemic and result in the patient presenting in a toxic state with a tachycardia. The plain radiograph is usually diagnostic.

(d) *Pseudo-obstruction.* In this condition the colon becomes distended and behaves as though obstructed, but there is no mechanical obstructing lesion. It is classified as primary, where there is a motility disorder, or secondary, where there may be an electrolyte or metabolic disorder, history of trauma or collagen disorder. An instant enema is important as laparotomy in these patients is contraindicated and may be detrimental. It is unusual for pseudo-obstruction to present with a mass.

(e) *Ischaemic stricture.* These lesions are rare and due to a disruption of the blood supply, and may follow an attack of ischaemic colitis. Acute ischaemia can resolve after an acute attack and this is the usual outcome. Stricture formation can occur some weeks after an acute episode and rarely gangrene can occur. It can be accompanied by systemic disturbance and toxicity. The rectal passage of blood and mucus as well as the presence of a tender mass may be found.

(f) *Inflammatory bowel disease.* Crohn's disease can cause large-bowel strictures, resulting in obstruction.

2. (a) *Investigations.* He will require baseline haematological and biochemical analysis.

A plain supine abdominal radiograph will indicate that obstruction is present but is not usually helpful in establishing the cause or site. An unprepared water-soluble enema (Gastrografin) may demonstrate the classical signs of an obstructing carcinoma (apple-core lesion with shouldering and little or no passage of contrast through the stricture), but often indicates the level of obstruction without diagnostic features.

(b) *Management.* Preoperative correction of any possible haematological or biochemical imbalance will be required. He will require urinary catheterization to assess his urine output. Nasogastric decompression is usually required preoperatively. In view of his age, a chest radiograph and electrocardiogram (ECG) should be arranged. Fully informed consent for surgery, explaining the possible need for a stoma, has to be obtained.

3. It is important to perform a thorough laparotomy and assess whether there is hepatic involvement, synchronous lesions in the colon and any evidence of peritoneal seedlings.

   The overall condition of the patient and resectability of the lesion must be evaluated when deciding on the type of operation. See Table 33.1 for the various surgical options.

   Decompression is the principal aim of the first operation. Whether or not resection should be carried out at the first operation and whether or not a primary anastomosis should be performed continue to be matters for debate.

   If the situation is not suitable for prolonged surgery, decompression can be achieved with a loop transverse colostomy, making sure to bring it out to the right of the middle colic vessels. Caecostomy is no longer used; it does not provide a total faecal diversion and can become dislodged and infected and is difficult for the patient to manage.

   Resection is preferable if the patient's condition allows. The patient can undergo a sigmoid colectomy with formation of an end stoma and distal mucous fistula. Alternatively the distal end can be closed and left in the pelvis (Hartmann's procedure), but this should be done only if the bowel wall is in a satisfactory state to take sutures or staples. Moreover a mucous fistula is easily identified during any subsequent operation to restore intestinal continuity.

Table 33.1 Operative possibilities for the colorectal case

Surgical principle	*Operative procedure*
Decompression	Colostomy

Resection without anastomosis	Sigmoid colectomy
	Subtotal colectomy
	  Hartmann's ± mucous fistula
	  Paul-Mickulicz

Resection with anastomosis	Colorectal anastomosis ± defunctioning stoma Ileorectal anastomosis ± defunctioning stoma

A double-barrelled colostomy, as described by Paul-Mikulicz, can be fashioned if the distal end can reach the anterior abdominal wall. This procedure has the advantage of subjecting the patient to one anaesthetic, as the double-barrelled colostomy is closed after the bowel has decompressed and the patient has recovered from the initial stages of the anaesthetic and operation, with the use of an enterotome. The mucosa, bowel wall and anterior abdominal wall close over the lumen spontaneously once the faeces are passing down into the rectum.

Immediate resection and anastomosis (colectomy with ileorectal or ileosigmoid anastomosis) can be performed. Many surgeons would perform this with a covering ileostomy. If there is gross obstruction, colonic lavage via the appendix stump may have to be performed. Routine appendicectomy is performed and a large Foley catheter is inserted through the appendix stump and secured with a pursestring suture. The resection is performed and the proximal end of the colon is either passed over the side of the wound in order to allow a kidney bowl to collect the irrigation fluid or else large tubing is secured to the bowel with sutures and passed into a bucket beside the operating table. Saline is irrigated through the catheter until the fluid is clear. This removes the proximal faeces, which could disrupt the anastomosis in the early stages of healing.

If synchronous lesions are felt to be present in the right side or transverse colon a subtotal colectomy should be performed. An ileorectal anastomosis can be performed at the same operation (with or without a covering loop ileostomy) or else the terminal ileum can be brought out as an endostomy and the anastomosis performed at a later stage.

4. A polyp is an abnormal elevation from an epithelial surface. It is derived from the Greek *polypus*, meaning many feet, and originally referred to the cuttlefish.

   Polyps are classified into neoplastic and non-neoplastic groups (Table 33.2).

5. There are several high-risk groups associated with colorectal cancer.
   (a) *Benign neoplasms: adenoma.* All colorectal cancers probably arise from adenomas; however, only a minority of adenomas become malignant. The ability of an adenoma to become malignant is known as its malignant potential. This is thought to be governed by the size of the lesion,

Table 33.2 Classification of polyps

Neoplastic	*Non-neoplastic*
Benign	Metaplastic (hyperplastic)
Adenoma*	
Tubular	Hamartomatous
Villous	Peutz–Jeghers
	Juvenile
Malignant	
Adenocarcinoma	Inflammatory
Rare epithelial malignancy	Crohn's
	Ulcerative colitis
	Amoebiasis
	Schistosomiasis
	Diverticulitis

* Polyposis syndromes: familial adenomatous polyposis, Gardner's syndrome and Turcot's syndrome.

histological type and degree of epithelial dysplasia and morphology. Malignancy is more likely in patients with multiple adenomas.

Adenomas less than 1 cm rarely become malignant, and about 25% of polyps greater than 2 cm diameter are likely to contain a malignant focus. Tubular (usually pedunculated) adenomas are far less likely to be malignant than villous (usually sessile) adenomas. Dysplasia is classically classified as being mild, moderate and severe. The malignant potential is greatest with severe dysplasia. Adenomas may have a familial prevalence (see below).

(b) *Familial.* About 20% of first-degree relatives of patients with large-bowel cancer will themselves develop the disease. In some cases it is possible to identify a pattern of inheritance. In these syndromes the adenoma is again the premalignant lesion.

(i) *Hereditary non-polyposis colorectal cancer (HNPCC).* There are families where an increased incidence of adenocarcinoma of the colon and endometrium and an early age of onset of these neoplasms have been described. There is also an increased incidence of other multiple primary neoplasms, including ovary and breast. The genetic defects are thought to be in chromosomes 2 and 17. These families require screening and counselling.

(ii) *Familial adenomatous polyposis (FAP).* FAP is caused by an autosomal dominant gene mutation with a high degree of penetrance in the general population. The incidence in the general population is around 1 in 10 000. The primary defect is on the long arm of chromosome 5, in what is now known as the APC gene. There should be more than 100 adenomas in the large bowel for FAP to be diagnosed, although gene analysis will give a precise diagnosis in so-called informative families. Gardener described a series of extra-gastrointestinal conditions which are associated with the condition and these include sebaceous cysts, osteomata of the skull, maxilla and mandible, and desmoid tumours. This condition is a variant of FAP.

Gastric, duodenal and small-bowel adenomas occur and there is an increased risk of periampullary malignant disease as well as thyroid cancer.

(c) *Chronic inflammation*

(ii) *Ulcerative colitis.* Ulcerative colitis is known to have a malignant potential. This is thought to be related to the duration of the disease rather than the age of onset and the anatomical extent of large bowel involved. Precancerous epithelial dysplasia often develops in a flat mucous membrane and may not be evident macroscopically. This makes detection difficult.

(ii) *Crohn's disease.* There is an increased risk of developing large-bowel cancer compared to the normal population. However, this risk is far less than that associated with ulcerative colitis.

(iii) *Schistosomiasis.* In areas where *Schistosoma mansoni* and *S. japonicum* are endemic, such as the Sudan and Egypt, inflammatory masses called bilharziomas are produced by retention of ova in the mucosa of the large intestine. An association with colorectal cancer has been demonstrated, in the same way that *S. haematobium* has been associated with bladder cancer.

Further reading

Phillips SF, Pemberton JH and Shorter RG. (1991) Large bowel cancer. In: *The Large Intestine*, 1st edn, Nicholls RJ and Phillips RKS (eds). Raven Press, New York, pp. 657–686

Williams NS. (1993) Surgical management of carcinoma of the colon and rectum. In: *Surgery of the Anus, Rectum and Colon*, 1st edn, Keighley MRB, Williams NS (eds) WB Saunders, London, pp. 886–938

Humphrey J. Scott
Christopher T.M. Speakman
R. John Nicholls

Case 34 Bleeding oesophageal varices and portal hypertension

A 55-year-old man with known alcoholic cirrhosis was admitted as an emergency with acute haematemesis and cardiovascular collapse. Clinical examination revealed the stigmata of cirrhosis and an enlarged spleen. After adequate resuscitation, an upper gastrointestinal endoscopy was performed; it revealed actively bleeding oesophageal varices.

Questions

1. What is the emergency treatment of acute variceal bleeding?
2. Describe injection sclerotherapy.
3. What are the hazards of injection sclerotherapy?
4. What are the results of acute injection sclerotherapy?
5. What are Child's criteria?
6. What pharmacological measures are available and how effective are they?
7. Describe the role and techniques of balloon tamponade, mentioning any complications.
8. What is the role of emergency surgery?
9. What would be the definitive treatment of a patient who has had variceal bleeding?
10. What is the role, if any, of prophylactic therapy in variceal bleeding?

Answers

1. Variceal bleeding *must* be confirmed on urgent upper gastrointestinal endoscopy, once the patient is adequately resuscitated, and must never be assumed just because the patient is cirrhotic. If there is doubt on initial endoscopy, endoscopy must be repeated within a few hours to obtain a better view. The choice of therapy depends on the severity of bleeding and whether the varices are easily visible on endoscopy. In the absence of severe haemorrhage

rendering the patient unstable, the current choice is a combination of injection sclerotherapy along with pharmacological agents which lower the portal venous pressure or constrict the lower oesophageal sphincter. Oesophageal tamponade is reserved for those patients who still bleed in spite of these measures or in whom the endoscopic view is insufficiently clear to allow accurate injection sclerotherapy.

2. Intravariceal injection is usually performed through a fibreoptic endoscope and less commonly through a rigid oesophagoscope (under general anaesthesia), especially if the varices are too bulky. The aim is to cause sclerosis or thrombosis of the varices and 5–6 ml of 5% ethanolamine is injected into each of three to four venous columns. An alternative technique is to inject sclerosant on either side (the paravasal technique) of the venous columns, following which fibrosis gradually compresses the varices. The intravasal technique is known to produce a quicker result.

   Injection schlerotherapy is a satisfactory technique in the presence of active haemorrhage but ideally the patient should first be resuscitated after balloon tamponade control of his haemorrhage so that the varices may be injected later and in the best possible conditions.

3. Injecting accidentally superficial to a varix will produce ulceration and the risk of secondary haemorrhage. A simple manometric device is available to confirm that the tip of the needle is neither too superficial nor too deep. Other serious complications include oesophageal stricture and perforation, pleural effusion and empyema. Minor complications include low-grade pyrexia, retrosternal discomfort and tachycardia.

4. A review of 25 years of acute sclerotherapy in Belfast showed a high rate of success, while major morbidity was uncommon. Oesophageal perforations in the series were the result of routine use of the rigid oesophagoscope. The 264 patients included in the review included both noncirrhotics and patients with extrahepatic causes of portal hypertension, while the overall mortality (mainly from liver failure and hepatorenal syndrome) was proportional to the severity, as determined by Child's criteria.

5. C.G. Child's prognostic classification of patients with chronic liver disease based on clinical and laboratory data

Table 34.1 Child's criteria for prognostic classification

Criteria	*Child's grade A*	*Child's grade B*	*Child's grade C*
Serum bilirubin (mmol/l)	< 34	23–57	> 51
Serum albumin (g/l)	35	28–35	< 28
Prothrombin time (in seconds prolonged)	1–4	4–6	> 6
Ascites	Absent	Slight	Moderate
Encephalopathy	None	Minimal	Coma

(1964) also allows the assessment of any interventional or operative risk.

Patients on Child's grade A have a 70% 1-year survival and the best chance of surviving elective and emergency surgery, with the prognosis worsening for those of grade B or C.

6. Vasopressin, which is a constrictor of the splanchnic circulation alone, is probably of little benefit and has the disadvantages of causing abdominal colic, a decrease in coronary and hepatic perfusion and an antidiuretic effect, causing fluid retention. Glypressin is longer-acting with fewer side-effects, but none of them can control more than half the patients with acute variceal bleeding and there is an unacceptably high recurrence rate. Vasopressin has also been known to cause cutaneous gangrene when given in infusion form (as opposed to bolus injections). On the other hand, it is especially useful in children with portal hypertension as it helps avoid balloon tamponade in the young.

   Other drugs which are helpful in conjunction with vasopressin are glyceryl trinitrate (which also lowers portal venous pressure), metoclopramide (which constricts the lower oesophageal sphincter and controls variceal bleeding) and somatostatin, whose action is unknown and is used only in the context of controlled clinical trials.
7. Tamponade is a life-saving measure in severe and uncontrolled variceal haemorrhage where pharmacological control is inappropriate and acute schlerotherapy impossible. The technique is safe when supervised and is a vital temporizing measure prior to transfer to specialist centres.

A standard technique involves the Minnesota modification of the Sengstaken-Blakemore tube which has two balloons and two suction channels. After pretesting the balloon, the tube is inserted nasally or orally and the gastric balloon inflated to at least 300 ml once the tube is well beyond the 40 cm mark from the incisor teeth. The balloon is pulled back against the cardia and the oesophageal balloon inflated to about 120 ml. Preinflating this balloon to even distension helps to measure this exact volume. The tube is then fixed to the patient's forehead, the oesophageal channel connected to continuous low-pressure suction to empty secretions and the gastric channel connected to continuous drainage. Balloon tamponade should not be used for more than 12 h continuously and 24 h in total to void the risk of pressure necrosis. A useful technique is to cool the tube in a refrigerator so as to stiffen it and make insertion easier.

In a review of 17 series, the control rate with balloon tamponade was 77%, but further bleeding occurred in 50% and half the patients subsequently died.

Complications include oesophageal ulceration and rupture, aspiration pneumonia, asphyxia and ulceration of the nares.

8. Half the patients with acute variceal haemorrhage will stop with vasopressin or tamponade and the majority who rebleed will be controlled by acute sclerotherapy. The place for emergency surgery is thus limited.

   Surgery is usually in the form of oesophageal transection with or without devascularization, the aim being to interrupt venous flow into the upper stomach and lower oesophagus. One must bear in mind that this is a large operation for very sick people, and carries significant morbidity and mortality.

   Emergency portocaval shunts, although most effective in preventing rebleeding, carry a high operative mortality and a prohibitive incidence of postoperative encephalopathy.
9. Once the acute bleeding is controlled, the patient must be assessed carefully for definitive treatment. The choice lies between a portosystemic shunt, transection with devascularization and chronic sclerotherapy.
   (a) *Selective portosystemic shunt* in the form of a distal splenorenal (Warren's) shunt has a place in the defini-

tive treatment of patients with Child's grade A or B_2 who are under 50 years of age and are not diabetic. The risk of rebleeding is minimal and the risk of postoperative encephelopathy and liver failure acceptably low in these patients. There is, however, no significant improvement in terms of survival.

(b) Oesophageal transection with devascularization may be useful in good-risk patients who are unsuitable for a shunt for whatever reason, but itself carries a 10% operative mortality and the risk of anatomical leakage, dysphagia, encephalopathy and an incidence of recurrent haemorrhage higher than that of a shunt. Trials are underway comparing this with long-term injection sclerotherapy.

(c) *Elective long-term sclerotherapy* at weekly intervals has been shown to be more effective and carry an increased survival than portosystemic shunting. It is certainly the treatment of choice for patients with jaundice, severe ascites, small liver size and poor liver function (i.e. Child's grade C) who would not tolerate laparotomy very well. Disadvantages include all the complications of injection sclerotherapy and the need for the patient to come regularly to hospital on a long-term basis.

10. There is no place for shunts in patients who have not bled from varices and several trials reported so far have shown no benefit in offering prophylactic sclerotherapy to these patients.

Further reading

Hamilton G. (1994) Oesophageal varices: aetiology, presentation and investigation. In: *Oxford Textbook of Surgery*, vol. 1, Morris PJ and Malt RA (eds). Oxford University Press, Oxford, p. 1252

Johnson AG and Taylor I. (1992) The liver and portal circulation. In: *The New Aird's Companion in Surgical Studies*, Barnard KG and Young AE (eds). Churchill Livingstone, Edinburgh, pp. 1097–1128

Spence RAJ and Johnston GW. (1986) Oesophageal varices: pathogenesis and management. In: *Recent Advances in Surgery*, vol. 12, Russell RCG. (ed.) Churchill Livingstone, Edinburgh, pp. 105–123

M. Sen

Case 35 Parotid gland tumour

A 40-year-old female presented to her general practitioner with a 5-year history of a lump in the neck. The patient was asymptomatic and had responded by growing her hair to cover the lump. Eventually she was coaxed to attend the doctor by her sister. Examination revealed a 2-cm-diameter round rubbery nodular lump a little in front and above the angle of the jaw on the right side. The patient was referred to surgical outpatients.

Questions

1. What is the most likely diagnosis and how would you clinically determine whether it was likely to be benign or malignant?
2. What other pathologies of the parotid gland can mimic neoplasia?
3. How do you classify parotid tumours?
4. What special investigations are available to confirm the diagnosis of a parotid tumour?
5. Outline the surgical steps for a superficial parotidectomy.
6. What complications may develop following superficial parotidectomy for pleomorphic adenoma?

Answers

1. Pleomorphic (mixed) salivary adenoma is the commonest tumour of the parotid gland and accounts for 55% of all parotid masses and 80% of benign parotid tumours. A typical history is of an asymptomatic mass for many years and the principal complaint is the existence of a mass. The vast majority of parotid tumours are sited in the superficial lobe (81%) in the region of the angle of the jaw. Tumours of the deep lobe will swell the parapharyngeal space and displace the tonsil. Intraoral and bimanual palpation of the tumour are therefore mandatory in the clinical assessment of a parotid tumour. The differential diagnosis for a lump in the region of the tail of the parotid includes:

(a) *Lymphadenopathy*, which may be localized or generalized, benign or malignant. Tuberculosis should always be considered, but a cold abscess is often tender.
(b) *Branchial cyst*. This embryological remnant of the pharyngeal pouch very uncommonly presents over the age of 40 years. Classically the swelling is sited on the anterior border of the sternocleidomastoid muscle and is fluctuant.
(c) *Cystic hygroma*. This congenital anomaly of the jugular lymph sac is usually manifest in early infancy.
(d) *Non-epithelial tumours*. These include lipoma, neurofibroma and haemangioma (commonest in childhood).
(e) *Vascular lesions*. Carotid artery aneurysm and chemodectoma should be considered.
(f) *Hypertrophy of the masseter* may be acquired from habitual grinding of the jaw (bruxism).

The two features indicative of a malignant parotid tumour are facial nerve paralysis and regional lymphadenopathy. Even the largest of benign tumours will not give rise to facial paralysis as the nerve becomes stretched over the slowly enlarging mass. However, very large tumours are more likely to be malignant.

2. A variety of non-neoplastic disorders may mimic a parotid tumour.
   (a) Acute infection (sialadenitis) can be either viral (mumps) or bacterial. Viral infections are common and may be epidemic. The less commonly encountered bacterial parotitis affects debilitated patients, those with poor oral hygiene and may follow head and neck radiotherapy.

   With the advent of better perioperative fluid balance, acute postoperative parotisis is rare. Clinically there is typically a brawny swelling of the entire parotid and pus may be expressed along Stensen's duct.
   (b) Salivary duct calculi may give rise to intermittent swelling of the gland, typically at the time of eating. Dehydration and poor oral hygiene predispose to salivary calculi. Secondary bacterial infection may occur. The diagnosis is made from the history, bimanual palpation of the duct and radiology (plain X-ray or sialography).
   (c) Chronic inflammation of the parotid occurs in patients with Sjögren's syndrome (sicca disease) manifest by xerophthalmia, xerostomia and connective tissue disease (e.g. rheumatoid arthritis) and in granulomatous

diseases, including tuberculosis and sarcoidosis. Therefore a general examination for the presence of systemic disease should always be performed.

3. Tumours of the salivary (parotid) glands may be benign or malignant, the latter primary or secondary.
   (a) *Benign*
      (i) *Pleomorphic salivary adenoma*, so-termed as the tumour comprises both epithelial and mesenchymal elements, is the commonest benign tumour (80%). It is well-encapsulated but pseudopod extensions of the tumour extend beyond the capsule. For this reason, simple enucleation of the tumour predisposes to a local recurrence rate between 25% and 50%. Conversely, adequate resection by means of a superficial parotidectomy has a recurrence rate closer to 1%. It is estimated that between 2% and 6% of tumours may undergo malignant transformation, this event being more common following local recurrence.
      (ii) *Adenolymphoma (Warthin's tumour)* accounts for 14% of benign parotid neoplasms. It is believed to arise from salivary glands that were embryologically located within a parotid lymph node and nearly all Warthin's tumours are located within the parotid. The tumour is well-encapsulated and malignant transformation is rare (0.3%).
      (iii) *Oxyphilic tumours (oncocytomas)* constitute 1% of benign parotid tumours and are seen in older patients.
   (b) *Primary malignant tumours* (25% of all parotid tumours)
      (i) *Mucoepidermoid carcinoma* is the commonest malignant tumour of the parotid (44%). It is typically slow-growing and favours local invasion, but facial paralysis is rarely seen.
      (ii) *Malignant mixed tumour* is believed by some to arise from pleomorphic tumours, but possesses the morphology of adenocarcinoma. Local lymph node involvement is seen in 25% of cases at presentation.
      (iii) *Acinic cell carcinoma* is often multilobular and commomer in females. Whilst it has the propensity for distant spread, local invasion is more usual.
      (iv) *Adenoid cystic carcinoma* is seen in 9% of malignant parotid tumours. These tumours are often slow-

growing, but perineural spread is typical and the extent of the disease is often clinically underestimated.

(c) *Secondary malignant tumours*
Malignant melanoma and *squamous cell carcinoma* are the commonest secondary deposits, of which 60% of the primary tumours are located in the head and neck. Other primary sites include lung, kidney and breast.

4. Fine-needle aspiration cytology (FNAC) may provide a cytological diagnosis, but is dependent upon the experience of the local cytopathologist. Whilst some centres advocate routine FNAC in all patients, others employ it selectively. Concurrence rates of 95% for benign and 85% for malignant lesions have been reported. FNAC is *least* accurate in diagnosing pleomorphic adenomas and mucoepidermoid carcinomas. FNAC may also be used in the assessment of lymph nodes and this may be of value in distinguishing inflammatory and neoplastic pathology.

   Small mobile tumours in the superficial lobe do not usually justify radiological assessment, which is reserved for those tumours which are fixed or located deep within the gland. Radiology, either by computed tomography (CT) or magnetic resonance imaging (MRI), provides greater detail regarding the position and extent of the tumour and its anatomical relationship to adjacent structures. In addition, MRI can directly image the seventh cranial nerve. Occasionally, MRI may provide a clue to the histological diagnosis of the tumour. Adenolymphomas produce a hot spot on technetium-99 isotope scanning.
5. The two cardinal objectives are preservation of the facial nerve and adequate tumour clearance. Under controlled hypotension and with the patient's head elevated, a skin excision is created in the preauricular skin crease commencing at the level of the zygoma, curving posteriorly around the ear lobe and turning inferiorly in the skin crease of the neck over the anterior border of sternocleidomastoid muscle. The incision is deepened through platysma and the greater auricular nerve is divided. Deeper dissection reveals the posterior belly of digastric muscle, the mastoid process and the external auditory meatus. The main trunk of the facial nerve is then exposed in the tissues between the cartilaginous auditory canal, the tip of the mastoid process and the superior border of the posterior belly of digastric

muscle. The exposure is facilitated by forward retraction of the parotid tissue. Using artery forceps and sharp dissection, a plane separating the superficial lobe of the salivary gland from the main trunk of the facial nerve and its divisions is created. The ultimate objective is to reflect forwards the parotid tissue away from the facial nerve until the anterior margin of the gland has been reached. Stensen's duct is finally identified, ligated and divided and the wound closed over a suction drain.

6. Following excision of a superficial parotid pleomorphic adenoma, the following complications may arise:
   (a) Haematoma is reported to occur in about 5% of cases, despite surgical drainage. This may in part reflect a reluctance to employ the diathermy for fear of facial nerve damage.
   (b) Facial nerve paralysis. Neuropraxia is seen in about 15% of cases. Patients should be warned preoperatively and frequently reviewed in the outpatient department. When the eyelid is affected, eyedrops should be prescribed and the patient advised to avoid exposure to the elements until full recovery. In the event of accidental division of the nerve, repair should be immediately attempted using a graft from either the greater auricular or sural nerves. A lateral tarsorrhaphy may be indicated. When permanent paresis results, a number of plastic surgical procedures are available to improve facial symmetry and function.
   (c) Salivary fistula formation is uncommon and usually resolves spontaneously with adequate drainage.
   (d) Frey's syndrome is characterized by flushing and sweating of the skin innervated by the auriculotemporal nerve whenever salivation is stimulated – so-called gustatory sweating. It is believed to arise secondary to a cross-wiring between secretomotor nerve fibres to the parotid gland (postganglionic parasympathetic fibres from the otic ganglion) and sympathetic nerves to the sweat glands of the skin in the preauricular region, following injury to the auriculotemporal nerve. Frey's syndrome becomes manifest within the first year of surgery and is typically self-limiting. In extreme cases intratympanic parasympathetic neurectomy is considered.
   (e) Local recurrence of the tumour is related to the adequacy of the primary dissection. Recurrences are

frequently multiple and involvement of the facial nerve is much more commonly encountered (eight times more often). Although secondary surgery is treacherous, a 10% rate of malignant transformation of recurrent benign tumours is reported. Re-excision of these tumours is therefore recommended, and some centres employ adjuvant radiotherapy. In some circumstances, when the recurrences are multiple or pose a significant risk to the facial nerve, radiotherapy alone may be considered. However, it should be noted that late local recurrences of tumour following radiotherapy are often malignant.

Further reading

Larsson SG. (1991) Comparison of methods of imaging the salivary glands. *Current Opinions in Radiology* **3:** 76–83

Lin FF, Rotstein L, Davison AT *et al.* (1995) Benign parotid adenomas: a review of the Princess Margaret Hospital experience. *Head and Neck* **17:** 177–183

Megarian CA and Maniglia AJ. (1994) Parotidectomy: a ten year experience with fine needle aspiration and frozen section biopsy correlation. *Ear Nose and Throat Journal* **73:** 377–380

Witten J, Hybert F and Hansen HS. (1990) Treatment of malignant tumours in the parotid gland. *Cancer* **65:** 2515–2520

David M. Scott-Coombes
John A. Lynn

Index

The page numbers in **bold** type refer to Figures or Tables

Printed in the United Kingdom
by Lightning Source UK Ltd.
9783800001BA/4